French Dressing

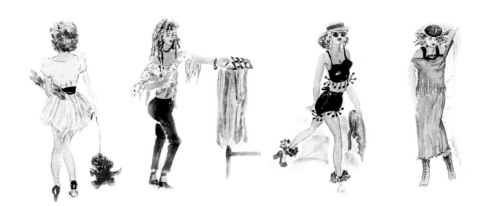

French Dressing with Italian seasoning
and the zest of two ripe lemons
Monica Matterson

Text © Monica Matterson
Illustrations © Monica Matterson
Design © 131 Design Ltd
www.131design.org

ISBN 978 1 909660 51 9

A CIP catalogue record for this book is available
from the British Library.

Published 2015 by Tricorn Books,
131 High Street, Old Portsmouth,
PO1 2HW

www.tricornbooks.co.uk

Printed & bound in UK

French Dressing

*with Italian seasoning
and the zest of
two ripe lemons*

Monica Matterson

Contents

Chapter 1	9
Chapter 2	14
Chapter 3	31
Chapter 4	36
Chapter 5	110
Chapter 6	139
Chapter 7	152
Chapter 8	178
Chapter 9	183
Chapter 10	195
Chapter 11	214
Chapter 12	224
Chapter 13	228

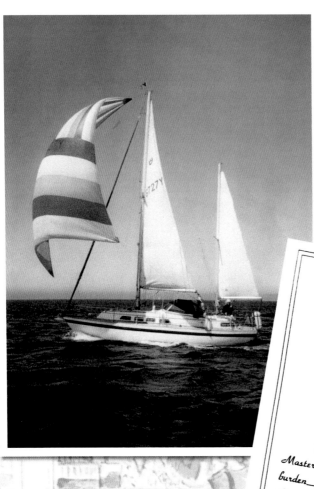

The United St

DEPARTMENT OF
UNITED STATES CU

CLEARANCE OF VESSEL

These are to certify all whe

That _CPT MATTESON_

Master or Commander of the _KALIVA_

burden_____ Tons, or thered

Guns, navigated with _TWO_ Men

FIBERGLASS built, and bound for _NASSO_

_____

_____

_____

with passengers and having on board _IN_

_____

MERCHANDISE AND ST

hath here entered and cleared his said vessel, according to

Given under our hands and seals, at the Customho

_____ , this _APR 5 1990_ day

on thousand nine hundred _90_ ,and in t

year of the Independence of the United States of America

Preface

Contrary to the impression given by the title, this is not a recipe book, but more of a strictly, non-educational drift through France and Italy with a retired couple in their 32ft ketch. It combines the sweet and sour taste of Mediterranean cruising with the hopes and fears of these two slightly timorous wrinklies while taking a poke at every day life and customs.

The narrative is woven round sketches made during the voyage with the observations being highly non-technical.

Since this time, conditions have greatly improved with the introduction of modern navigational aids, radar and mobile telephones to make passaging much simpler for the would-be cruisers. There are also many more new modern marinas now.

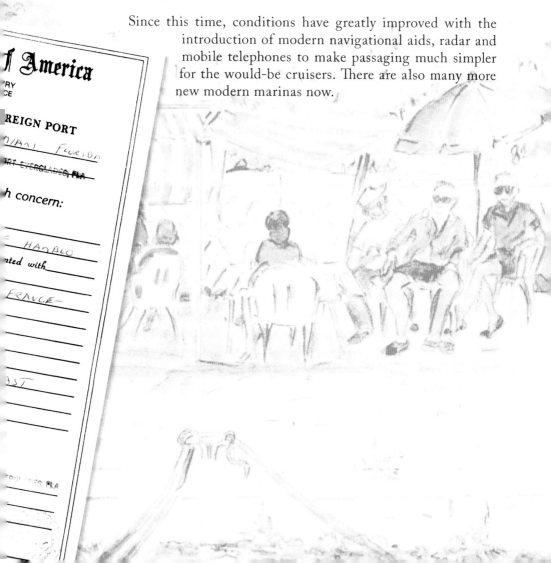

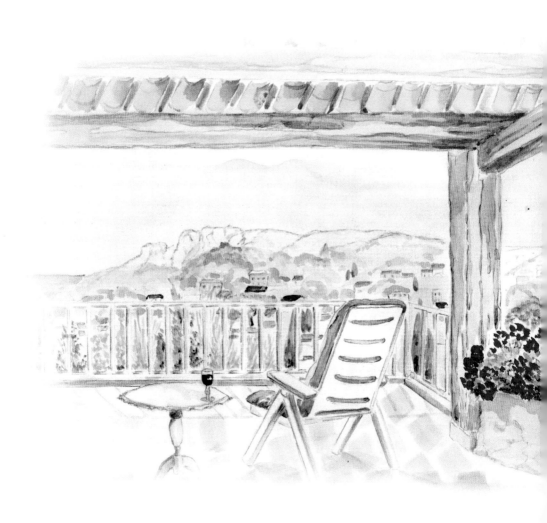

Balcony at Cassis

Chapter one

Battered light twists

The year is 1990, in the month of May. Our 32ft Finnish built ketch, *Kalivala* is somewhere in the mid-Atlantic on a cargo ship en route from Fort Lauderdale in Florida to Marseilles. My husband Sam, is also crossing the Atlantic on a Sparkman Stevens 68ft ketch, *Olivia* – with four colleagues. He retired, supposedly, earlier this year from a medical manufacturing company in Florida, but is now counted as a consultant and is therefore still occasionally beholden to his ex-employer, Carl, who owns this beautiful sleek yacht, named after his fourth wife!

Meanwhile, I am busy languishing in a pretty villa overlooking the picturesque bay of Cassis in Provence, anxiously awaiting their return. This three-story villa is rented by Carl for the use of staff and visiting clients, usually doctors, yet it is very sparsely furnished on the vast expanse of ceramic-tiled floors. To compensate, the view from the long, wide balcony is so stunning that all you really need is a deck-chair and a table. The only other occupant at present is a secretary, Denise, who drives daily to La Ciotat, a few miles away, to the offices where Carl has set up a subsidiary company for European sales. To occupy myself in between trips to the beach and lolling on the balcony, I take on a few house-keeping duties which entail lugging the daily shopping up a hundred and twenty steps, and cooking supper.

One day, I did try to tidy the much overgrown garden, but the enthusiasm faded after unearthing some very weird creatures resembling see-through crickets while I was moving some rotten logs from the aggressive, eye-level nettles. These lovely May days seem so long, and very hot. I am concerned for the safety of *Olivia* and her crew, and am still waiting for news of the arrival of our own boat, *Kalivala* into Marseilles, while also becoming a little impatient to begin our own adventures.

After leaving Florida we had promised ourselves to sail down the Mediterranean sea, visit the famous sites in Rome, Pisa, Pompeii and Florence then move on to Greece, Turkey and onwards for as many years as we wished … and it is now into May with all this perfect weather going to waste. Then at last, I have news – *Kalivala* has arrived and is in a compound awaiting delivery and I am to be taken to see her the next day.

Sparsely furnished - all mod cons!

What an awful shock. The mast steps are buckled, the mast and stern lights are broken, the radar reflector is split and the wind-screen is shattered in its bent and broken frame. Tears prickle my eyes, blotting out the scene.

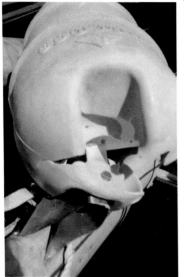

When *Kalivala* was shipped from England to Florida four years ago, we were not allowed to put any protective covering over her and didn't understand why. On *Kalivala's* return from Fort Lauderdale to the UK, we asked about this and were answered with a shrug and, "Sure you can, Ma'am!" So, in view of the filthy state *Kalivala* had arrived in at Fort Lauderdale, we decided to try and keep her as protected as possible. We put on the winter tarpaulin for the return passage. How wrong we were. It was a rough passage, and the seas broke over all the deck cargo, filling the top of our cover, creating a pond. The weight of it eventually caused the collapse of the wind-screen supports and the glass. We now know the reason why covering was not originally permitted!!

Damage to radar reflector

With help from the Ciotat office, I manage to sort out the tricky insurance claim forms and assessments to be ready for Sam's return, and also make arrangements for transporting and putting in the water at La Ciotat marina. To obtain a berth at the marina, Carl has to apply to the Mayor for special permission to stay whilst carrying out the repairs, for which we are most grateful.

On June 6th we have news that *Olivia* has blown into Porto Sherry in a force 7 storm. All crew are unscathed, although Sam had been washed down the deck a few times!

July 1st 1990 Bandol

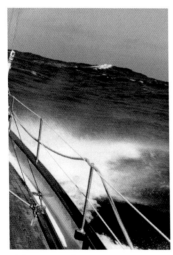

It is very emotional and a great relief for the friends, relatives and myself to catch sight of the full sails gradually nearing the harbour then, at last, taking down the sails to motor her into berth after the thirty-day crossing. The appropriate celebrations popped several corks before a very happy dinner party at the nearest restaurant.

Back at the villa, the weary crew enjoy the comfort of a bed that does not roll and that there are no watches to keep. For a more festive impression, I graced the table with a few flowers in a beer bottle!

Atlantic swell

After two days of rest and re-orientation it is now time to face the reality of repairing our own boat to make ready for our venture. The great excitement and anticipation of setting off almost immediately now fades with the thought of all the work yet to be done. As soon as *Kalivala* is back in the water, we move out of the villa to live aboard, thinking this would save time and travel. Quotes are made and a workman comes to undertake the screen repairs. The rest we can replace for ourselves, so there should only be a few more days before we will be ready to leave - so I thought! We are again elated, enthusiastic and full of ideas and plans for the places we wish to explore.

July 3rd 1990 Deflation

The local chandlers manage to supply all the necessary replacements; work progresses well and excitement grows. What we had not reckoned on were the whims of Carl! To understand a little of his personality, one needs to know that he is from the alliance between Basque and Cuban families. He is an astute and ruthless businessman, prone to sudden violent rages and is sometimes peevish but, he is also very generous, adventurous, ruggedly tall, handsome and a bit of a pussy cat. He has also given us some great experiences and a livelihood when Sam's own business went pear-shaped over four years ago, so Sam is very loyal to him, even at his most annoying times. I am not always so tolerant, though still grateful. Carl now starts by wanting a bit of help with some business matters, then, before long, we have been lent a company car and Sam is back in an office nearly every day, while I am left to fume a little and amuse myself all day on the boat. This I do by people-watching, observing, and making a few sketches and watercolours.

La Ciotat

This medium size, ordinary town lies between Marseilles and Toulon. It was once a thriving boat-building port producing methane gas tankers, but by 1990 the rusting cranes hang their heads over the derelict work-sheds midst the weeds that hide the broken glass from their empty window frames. The sight is depressing, but, once past the ancient disused *pissoir* and wash house, there is now a nature park where the elusive cicadas noisily rasp their chorus. Beyond are the *calanques*, rocky narrow inlets with sandy coves at the foot of the steep cliffs. The town centre is mainly a pedestrianised street of small shops leading downhill to the old port where the disgruntled out-of-work shipbuilders congregate outside the bars. On Tuesdays, a lively market throngs the streets where chickens roast on spits, vast pans of paella bubble, orientals try to sell you belts with rusty buckles, tortoises fall off their table and land upside down, and *escargots* escape from a wooden box to wander across the pavement. Meanwhile, Peruvian pan-pipes battling with their own version of *The Albatross* all help to add some character to the town.

The Great Escape

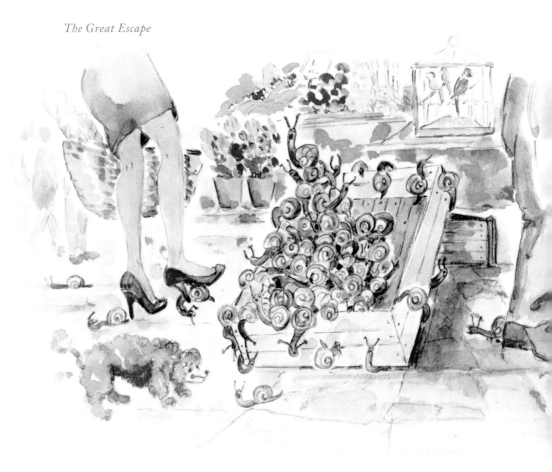

Run for it René. Now Pierre. Look out Claude! Poor Claud

One day, outside the vegetable shop at the top of the hill, there are some fresh looking cauliflowers. 'Make a nice change,' I thought, 'but what a lot of big leaves. They're not all necessary, especially as it is sold by weight!' Being Yorkshire by birth, I am not exactly mean but just very careful with money. I reckon that two or three less large outside leaves should make a bit of difference to the price, but not to the shape. Discreetly, I remove them and drop them back into the box before taking it inside to pay. Madam weighs it … 8 francs, 30 cents, then eyes it suspiciously before marching outside to bring in the giant discarded leaves to throw them defiantly on to the scales with the cauliflower. The price is now 12 francs. Those useless leaves cost nearly half as much the whole vegetable! My vocabulary blanks out not knowing how to say the French equivalent of "Get knotted" at short notice and I just manage a polite, quiet, *"Non, merci,"* before making what I thought to be a dignified exit.

Walks to the beach every day to swim are becoming a bit too routine, and one Sunday we find the equivalent of a church bazaar outside the cemetery and learn that it is in aid of the charity for stray cats and is taken very seriously here. The money raised goes to buy food for the dozens of feral felines that patrol the rocks round the harbour. Since they help to keep down the over-population of rats, the citizens of La Ciotat like to show their gratitude, but for us the walk round the cemetery has more appeal. It is sad to see how much some of the sentry box graves have been vandalised.

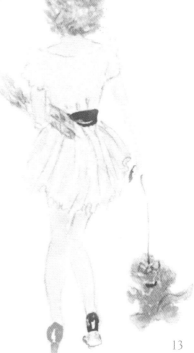

"Stop. Why are we wasting our time like this? We are supposed to be sailing."

There and then a sudden decision is made. To escape from Carl's demands we will go home for a month, tidy the garden and be around for the birth of our third grandson. (Sorry Carl.)

Chapter 2

First course

Actiivation. La Ciotat to St Mandrier and Isle de Porquerolle

September 19ᵗʰ 1990

I can hardly believe it! We are at last leaving La Ciotat today after a three and a half month delay. There is blue sky and sun but no wind, only the promise of a mistral later. All three sails are hoisted in hope of finding a capful of wind, but no, we have to succumb to the motor for the whole of the twenty two miles into the small port of St Mandrier within the bay of Toulon, which is grimly guarded by three old and rusting naval vessels. Once past these there is a small sheltered marina, a few bars and shops on the quayside, not highly exciting but we have at last made a start - and it only costs 70 francs per night. (About £7 at the time.)

The next day, the plan is to sail to the small Island of Porquerolle, just 12.5 miles away. Again, there seems to be no wind in the bay of Toulon but there is an obvious swell that was not there yesterday. By the time we reach the open sea, this and the wind have noticeably increased and, coming from the starboard quarter, makes a most uncomfortable motion. A radio call gives a few moments of light relief.

"Can zumbody 'elp me, pliz?"
"Ici Toulon Radio. . .que'st que vous voulez?" (What do you want?)
"Vil zumbody spik Inglish, pliz?"
"Ow can we 'elp you?"
"I 'av seen zumzing."
"Wat is problem? Wat is it wat you see? Wat is you position?"
"I see ze white smok in ze sky, und zen big splash in vater be'ind my boat.
My pozishun iss per'aps four zree noth und zix east. I tink."
"Ooooh, you are in pro'ibited military firing area !!"
"YA?? . . .Vel 'ow vas I to know??"

Poor man. We assume he altered course.

As we ourselves change course to pass between the islands, the sea calms slightly, but since the sea looks too disturbed for comfort in the anchorage, we blow into the marina on Porquerolle just in time for lunch.

When the *Capitainerie* re-opens at 3pm, we pay 110 francs for a breezy berth, which tosses all boats in the increasing wind, making white horses in the marina. The towering black clouds, which we assume to be advancing weather, are in fact, fires raging on the mainland near Le Lavandou, said to be started by bored, unhappy firemen!

There is no chance to sail next day with a force 9 gusting through every few minutes like an express train through a station – the Mistral. Cycling with difficulty up hill, we find the old Napoleonic fort which houses an interesting collection of artefacts brought up from the many wrecks in this area, and date back to Roman times, around 300BC. The view from the top is literally breath-taking; you can hardly breathe for the wind! Next, comes another climb. Pushing the bikes up a rough, steep path we come to the lighthouse, only to find a notice pinned to the door - *Fermé. Au reason du vent.* (Closed because of the wind.) So now back to the boat to watch the bedraggled participants of a local yacht race limping back with jammed furling gear, foresails in shreds and one flying his tattered spinnaker like an out-sized battle pennant. It is going to be a noisy night!

There is no abatement the next day, and our reading matter has become confined to the dictionary, the Bible and the backs of packets, until Anne from the catamaran kindly brings across some old magazines, which are swapped with our out-dated newspapers.

Food prices here are noticeably more expensive and the choice more limited. It is a pleasant little island with pine and eucalyptus trees, sugar canes and sandy beaches. In spite of day trippers arriving by the frequent ferry load, it is really quite unspoilt. There are only a few battered cars, an ancient, dented coupé taxi that is black, rusty and covered in dust, and hundreds of bicycles! This, again could have changed by now.

September 24th Porquerolle to Le Lavandou

The *Capitaine's* warning of another Mistral coming prompts us to leave early for this short passage, as Mistrals are not supposed to start in the mornings. Thus, there was not enough wind to fill the sails until the last two miles of the 11.5 mile distance. Here is a good marina for 87 francs per night, and only a short pace from the

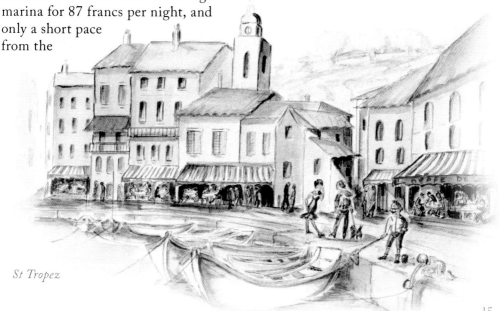

St Tropez

attractive shops, restaurants, quaint streets and beach, all explored in the afternoon before picking up a bottle of wine for 8 francs (80p). We dare not buy more in case it is like paint-stripper, but it does prove to be very drinkable. One slight disadvantage here, is the piped music which blares out from the top of every other lamp post along the promenade.

The forecast is now saying wind force 8-9, locally 10 with a very rough sea! What has happened to the weather since setting off? This decides us to cycle to Bormes Les Mimosas instead of an afternoon sail. The pert little girl in the Tourist Office says it is only 2 kilometres and not too steep. I did intend to go back later to tell her how wrong she was. However, this delightful village, over 2,000 years old in parts, is well worth every pint of sweat that the 6 kilometres and one in four hill to the top produces. When rested and quenched, the tourist path route leads up and down alleyways and countless steps where bougainvillea, roses, and geraniums tumble over the mellow stone parapets, and where through ancient archways are surprise glimpses across the lovely surrounding hills. The descent is almost painless, it just makes our arms and hands ache gripping the brakes!

September 25th St Tropez

"Happy birthday, Sam!" Let's go to St Tropez at 9.30am. At that remark the sky becomes very black and waves get bigger. After an hour sailing under jib and mizzen, we see where the fires are still smouldering right down to sea level near Cap Negrè having caused much devastation to forestry and houses. Ten miles down the coast, the radio gives out a Pan-pan call, warning all ships to look out for a stray, bleeping radio beacon. We look, but neither see nor hear it. How can they lose a thing like that? Once past Cap Camaret there is more shelter, so giving a good sail past *Cavaliere* and then, after 23 miles we turn into St Tropez at 3.30pm. It is now accepted as quite normal that *Sod's Law* is at work to send that sudden freak wind just as you enter a harbour and wish to look efficient. A slight fracas ensues involving rudders, and anchor chains. Since there are no pontoons, you have to drop anchor then reverse into a narrow slot up to the wall while fending off on all quarters and trying to look nonchalant. The 103 francs fee per night is more reasonable than expected. By now, there should be pontoons.

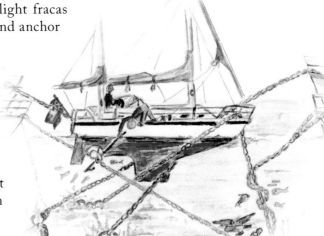

September 26ᵗʰ St Tropez to St Maxime

This morning we stroll through the town to admire the window displays of the delicatessens, patisseries and boutiques with eye-raising fashions at unbelievable prices. A steep climb up the hill to the citadel presents lovely views across the Gulf of St Tropez and the start of a yacht race. It includes some famous named boats like *Rothmans*, *Merit* and *Safilo,* which was called *Steinlager* in the Whitbread race.

Back at the old harbour, the sun glints through our beer glasses via reflections from the expanse of brass and mahogany of the elegant schooner opposite which is flying a red ensign. It is *Shenandoah*, owned by a renowned Round the World yachtsman. Its crew, or passengers, are just being collected for lunch by a uniformed chauffeur! We return for our baguette and pâté.

The gentle afternoon breeze tempts us to sail across the Gulf to St Maxime, just two miles away. By the time we arrive the breeze has become wind, which blows us hard onto the fuel dock. The *Capitaine* here is a Mademoiselle who helpfully tries to push away the boat ahead but has the misfortune to over-reach, resulting in some very spectacular contortions whilst dangling helplessly between two boats.

Grabbing her by the shirt, she just misses a ducking by a few inches, then with a swinging kick, and a heartfelt *"Mon Dieu!"* she manages to hook her legs over the pulpit to be dragged on board. It is with great dignity she, at last, serves our fuel. We do try not to laugh.

St Maxime is a very pleasant little town with quaint narrow streets, useful shops, a small museum, fountains, and a beach. Being conveniently moored next to the new shower block and 'Launderette', we pay for another night - 73 francs (about £7) seems reasonable.

There are quite a few English people to chat with, two being from our own home yacht club. Later, we are lulled to sleep by *Pierre* and his passionate love songs at a nearby restaurant. There is always some kind of night noise, if not, the security lights stream down the hatch and across your bunk.

September 28ᵗʰ St Maxime to St Raphael

How is it that whichever direction you wish to sail, the wind drops or shifts to a head wind? The sea is glassy calm and we motor the nine miles along the coast to the old port of St Raphael, which is said to be cheaper than the two new marinas. It is. The *Capitaine* is on holiday and we are shown into the space normally occupied by a pleasure boat that is away for repairs. A cycle ride into the old town proves it to be more 'tatty old' than 'interesting old' so the next day we ride the three miles up into Fréjus, which has much more character. Here is a Roman aqueduct, amphitheatre, city walls and gates, dating back to the first and second century. The cathedral has a fifth century baptistery; a proper guide is really needed but they only speak French. Free wheeling most of the way back down leaves enough time for a swim, although the sea is now becoming noticeably cooler.

Back in the cockpit, people-watching, glass in hand, we are interrupted by a slight diversion when a little boy loses his skate board over the dock side beside us. Not being quick enough with our long fishing net, the board slowly sinks the three metres to the bottom whilst the boy howls, and father scolds! By lashing our extending boat hook to the end of the fishing net, the board can just be touched if Sam hangs head first down while I hold his legs. One by one, interested passers by gather to watch, and after two or three gasping near-misses the skate board is duly retrieved amid much applause from the spectators and a "*Mercie beaucoup*" from its owner. The boy's father now carries the board as he prods the boy along the quayside as if to say, "Don't do that again."

September 30th Theoule sur mer

It is a dull, grey day, no wind, typical of when you decide to move on. In drizzle, we have to motor for the thirteen miles along the coastline of impressive high red cliffs, then creep slowly between rocks to look at Figuerettes. Too much modern construction! Next comes Galere Marina, all new with strange lopsided apartment blocks and looking deserted. Perhaps it is not yet finished? "Give it a miss, Sam!"

Continuing on to Theoule we find the very narrow, shallow entrance which appears to be almost on the beach. No one is there, so we tie up on the fuel jetty to go and look for the *Capitaine*. The office is closed and he is not in the bar – we check! The fuel pumps remain closed, we realise it is Sunday, so we stay.

The little town will be quite pleasant when the sun shines. Some locals are playing a noisy game of boules and others sedately parade in their finery along the water side path, which is dedicated to a past mayor. Much of this place resembles a miniature railway layout, it is on the mainline to Nice, with trains rattling through with persistent regularity. At night time the cliffs and the small castle are floodlit, the harbour entrance lights blink down into our cabin, and all is calm - until the next train!

The next day, sailing is cancelled. We locate the *Capitaine* as he walks his dog in the rain, pay him for a proper berth with electricity, and just finish tying up in time for a torrential downpour in a goodly thunderstorm which had blacked out Nice an hour ago.

October 2nd Cannes

Leaving early, we drift slowly along the coast for five miles under just jib and mizzen sails, and into Cannes, a much larger stop over than we prefer. I'm not sure I like it. The *Capitanerie* is so far away that we have to cycle round to check in. Surprise!! It is the cheapest mooring yet at 90 francs for two nights. I think we are warming to the place a little!

Cannes is lively and bustling, the shop windows artistically displayed and if you can afford the prices, there is no need to cook. Strangely, a bottle of beer, Coke or tonic costs more than wine, so we are revising our preferences!

October 3rd

It is grey and overcast, more like England than the Cote d'Azure so we catch a bus from near the Mairie (town hall) up to Grasse, which is yet another hilltop Medieval town famous for its perfumeries since the early 1700's. The companies of Fragonard, Molinard and Fleurras each have two factories here. As Fragonard is nearest to the bus stop, there we enjoy an interesting guided tour spoken in English which, of course, finishes at the gift shop. A few advance Christmas presents are settled before coming away lighter in purse, but smelling very much sweeter.

Most of the narrow streets are charming, but some parts are quite dilapidated and scruffy, making it hard to imagine that people really live there. The church holds a few antiquities including two large Reuben's paintings and, nicely timed, a trumpeter and organist are reverberating in exultation.

The bus returns us into the midst of another lively thunderstorm.

October 4th Precipitation

Our intention had been to leave today, but by ten o'clock the light rain has become heavy. With a bag of returnable bottles (every cent counts), in one hand and an umbrella in the other, my leap ashore is a near disaster when my foot hits   the wet metal strip on the pontoon. If you can imagine Mary Poppins landing flat on her back, still holding her bag and umbrella! No breakages luckily, but with a banged head and very bruised rump I hobble and slither, with Sam, round to the *Capitaine* to ask for another night's mooring.

In my best school French I wryly say, "*Je pense que nous ne voulons pas partir aujourd'hui.*" (I don't think we wish to leave today.) The *Capitaine* smiles, looks out of his window, and in perfect English replies, "Why not?" By this time yet another thunder storm is in full flash and his doormat is afloat, so we take as long as possible to pay before making a dash for the supermarket. At least it is dry inside, but they only accept the small bottles for return so, laden with empty and full ones, sundry edibles and a soggy baguette, we wade back. The streets are awash, and as we pass the now deserted little shops with their attractive displays, we reflect on the smells of France. Lavender, Rosemary, Pine and Eucalyptus trees, perfume, patisseries, flower markets, roasting chickens, fish, drains, toilets and dog dirt. So far, we are not exactly sure that this is classed as having a wonderful time.

October 5th

In spite of the sunny, blue morning, we pay for another night. Is this the onset of insidious port rot?

Today we cycle round to La Croisette, some rose gardens, an ornate Russian Orthodox Church and the Casino, by the side of which is an area of pavement adorned with the hand prints of film stars Meryl Streep, Jane Fonda, Rex Harrison, along with numerous unknowns. Here one mingles with the elite and the pigeons to survey the passing scene from the depth of a comfortable, free chair. There is more of interest in Cannes than first thought, as well as cheap moorings, so I must stop moaning.

October 6th To Antibes

There can be no more excuses today, although there is not much wind as we leave Cannes to motor-sail between Ile StMarguarita and Pt de la Croisette. A sudden drop in the depth, from 60ft to 12ft, causes temporary panic because the water is so crystal clear that it looks as if the keel is almost on the sea-bed. It takes nearly four hours to cover the ten miles to Antibes, but then, what is the hurry?

On entering the port, we call at the wrong *Capitanerie* first, among all the 100ft power boats I thought it didn't look quite 'us'. It is a vast marina, I am not impressed … too big, too impersonal, too costly, and our electric plug does not fit theirs. Then we realise it is on the flight path to Nice airport with planes landing every two minutes! There are many British boats here, but none as humble as *Kalivala*.

The town does prove to be more interesting with old ramparts, a 12th century cathedral, Picasso museum and a bustling square with its gaudy carousel.

Within the narrow old streets we are swept along in a wedding party then become trapped between hundreds of panting, sweating, Lycra'd charity supporters on their marathon run.

I get so bored sitting on this wall!

October 7th Antibes to Villefranche

Next day, the mild contention between us regarding whether we leave or stay is solved on our return from the market, by the man we come upon removing our mooring lines. He complains that we are in his place. On showing him our receipt with the dock number on, he apologises, we agree to leave and he dashes off to sort out the *Capitaine*, who possibly back-pocketed our 98 francs.

As usual, the few knots of breeze is *on the nose* but, not being in a hurry, we make a few long tacks, which brings us disconcertingly close to the airport runways which are so close to water's edge that you can wave to the passengers as they land!

A brief look into Nice harbour decides us against it, and so we sail on across the *Bai des Anges* for a further 11 miles into the attractive town of Villefranche. The harbour is small, the office is closed because it is Sunday, we see no spaces, so make fast in a grotty work area under the crane, and hope that we are not in anyone's way until Monday.

The town and its surrounds are enjoyable. We stay for six days, finding a better than average 15th century citadel housing five free museums of artwork and sculptures. There is a lively Sunday flea market and vivid flower gardens holding yet more sculptures by Volti, (he has a penchant for voluptuous women).

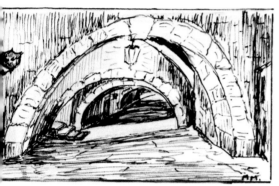

Rue Obscura, Villefranche

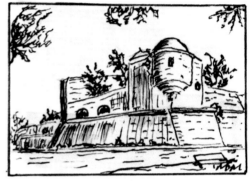

Citadel

One street of particular interest is the very old Rue Obscura, which leads below ground to tunnelled alleys with yet more art galleries.

Diversions

One town that we have organised for Poste Restante is Monte Carlo, just a short train journey away. Leaving Villefranche at 9.15am and carrying the usual bagful of empty bottles for return at a nearby little shop, we find said shop closed. Not wishing to tote them around all day, we line them up on the doorstep and continue a further mile to the station. The twenty minutes of fine coast-line and tunnels gives a glimpse of the main Monte Carlo marina where the huge opulent power boats are bucking crazily as big rollers pile in.

"We can give that one a miss." A long hike to the post office yields one welcome letter, promptly read before catching a bus up to the small Principality of Monaco. We arrive in the Palace Square just in the time for the changing of the Guard - all very smart in their drill uniforms and fancy hats, the scene is suggestive of the chorus in an operetta. The Palace did not look old or very interesting, but a 50 franc gamble on a guided tour in English proves us wrong. The reception rooms are richly decorated and have beautiful inlaid marble floors dating back to the 15th century.

Whilst trying to find our way back down again on foot, we come across the impressive cathedral. Inside are still the sad, drooping remains of the many elaborate wreaths left there after the recent funeral of Princess Caroline's husband Stephano, who was killed in a boating accident.

On the way back, the man in the shop laughs very loudly when we ask if he had found our bottles. "The man who lives upstairs cashed them in at 9.30am," he chuckles.

October 13ᵗʰ

At the top of a high sheer escarpment behind the harbour stands Fort Mont Alban which looks worth a visit, but it also looks to be a forbidding trek. Advised by the girl in the tourist office, we catch a minibus which fails to put us down at the right place. *"Pardon, pardon,"* says the driver. And so we get

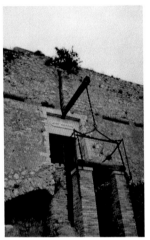 an interesting and spectacular extra drive to the bus terminus at Plateau St Michel, three peaks away from where we wish to be. Whilst waiting for the next bus to return, we oblige a couple of tourists by taking

their photographs, and they in return offer to give us a lift back – that is a big mistake. She is French, and drives dementedly round the hairpin bends; he is an attorney from Orlando. Somehow we arrive in Nice!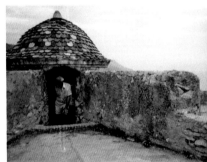

After stopping four times to ask the way we eventually come to a halt up a narrow rocky incline and having thankfully bid adieu, walk up the steps to Fort Mont Alban. It is in a hazardous state of disrepair, although the small drawbridge still works. Sam proves it by tipping me up. Numerous dark tunnels and precarious steps lead out onto the roof to fabulous views along the coast and hills; and there is our boat in the marina just below!! It is rather sad to see this castle so neglected and in such a dangerous condition. We walk down through a steep rocky forest path, with steps completely broken away in parts, to reach the road. Had we known, it would not have taken 25 miles to get there when it was only 1.5 miles to return.

October 11ᵗʰ

There follow three days of non events. Carl has organised to take Sam to the Genoa Boat Show, so its an early rise to get him spruced up and ready waiting. 9.30am, still waiting and waiting. On ringing the Ciotat office, Carl's secretary said he had left at 9.30am. Wait, wait. Ring again at 3pm and the secretary said, "I guess he's forgotten." I felt very cross and disappointed for Sam... a whole day wasted trying to stay clean - perhaps he'll come tomorrow, but who knows with Carl.

Not keen to waste another day, Sam disappears down the cockpit locker to cajole the 'Wallis' heater for the umpteenth time. I am in the shower when the water pump burns out, so Sam changes over to manual pump but then the tap leaks into the fridge. This is not the ideal time to be asked by the *Capitaine* to change places to further along the seawall because our electricity and water hose have the wrong connections. At least, Sam makes a perfect reverse into the new space. Funny sort of a day... then it rained!

The water pump is in pieces on the breakfast table the next day but is now functional, so Sam descends again into the locker trying to frighten the heater into submission, but to no avail.

We must move on tomorrow before *harbouritis* gets too firm a hold. For the last few days the night noises have been just distant, tolerable - accordion music from the bistro.

October 15th

The weather forecast is not good - thunder storms again and wind expected by afternoon; an early departure is made. Only 3 knots of wind with a 6ft swell does not make a comfortable sail but the 5.5 miles of coastline around Cap Ferrat is pleasing. After paying 80 francs for diesel fuel at Beaulieu Marina, we moor up on the visitors pontoon, where we are immediately ambushed by an over-zealous, sour faced customs official. He speaks no English, but I gather we are getting the third degree about our dates of arrival in France. He brandishes some forms before us. I ask, "*pour quoi?*" (why), he answers, "*parce-que*" (because) and then we realise that we are only 10 days off our allotted 6 month's stay in France. He is duly appeased by the completed forms which he stamps which a triumphant flourish and looks very pleased with himself.

The clouds are gathering and the Harbour Office can only allow one night at a time. Later we are visited by an English ex-naval commander on an old motorbike who is trying to sell us some admiralty charts. "No thanks, we have a tourist road map." The thunder rumbles and the next morning it is raining again; no point in sailing today.

First we check the cupboards for leaks, then suitably waterproofed we set out to explore our surroundings. The Van Gogh exhibition is closed, as is the Greek Museum - because it is Tuesday? We keep on walking around the bay past the casino, colourful gardens and attractive villas. An uphill climb brings us to a large pink and white confection of Isle de France, a beautiful villa once owned by Madame Ephrussi de Rothschild, which is now a museum of her treasures. The 35 francs entry fee each is well spent, even to just come in from the rain.

What a fascinating collection! There are well worn carpets and tapestries from the Vatican and the Palace of Versailles, writing desks said to once belong to Madame du Barry, Madam Pompadour and Marianne Antoinette. One set of carved doors came from an old chapel, apparently Madame de Rothschild had to buy the whole chapel just to get the doors. Many of the items are a bit threadbare or broken – I think she had scavenged round some very high ranking dustbins.

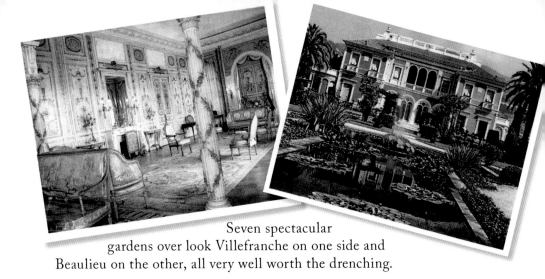

Seven spectacular gardens over look Villefranche on one side and Beaulieu on the other, all very well worth the drenching.

October 17ᵗʰ Beaulieu to Cap d' Ail, Monte Carlo

Sunshine! Clean shorts and shirts ready to take the train to Monte Carlo again. As we stop to pay for another night in the marina we are told, "The sun is shining, the sea is flat, you go." Having no choice, we leave with the wind on the nose, of course, and a slight swell for the 4 miles of grand coastline with the old village of Eze clinging to a peak.

The Cap d'Ail Marina, near Monte Carlo is not impressive, being surrounded by ongoing new development, but it is much more sheltered than Monte Carlo, so there we moor. A short scary cycle ride through a tunnel of zooming traffic takes us to the Post Office again where letters are waiting; it's great to have news from the family and friends.

The casino is an impressive, ornate building both inside and out but we get no further than the foyer. The 'heavies' wish us to leave our coats in the cloakroom or it is no entry. Adjacent to the casino, are the *Cafe du Paris* and the *Hotel du Paris* - such opulence - and we are not dressed for those either! The nearby streets are full of shops such as *Lanvin, Givenchy, Dior, Cartier, La Roche, Yves Saint Laurent* and a *Sotherbys* but, could we find a shop that sold meat or vegetables? I think everyone must eat out here. Another full-bodied thunderstorm serves as a lullaby and I tell myself yet again, 'This IS fun!'

October 18ᵗʰ

When heavy back clouds hang shrouding the mountains, and my washing hangs dripping over the guard rails, then it is a sure signal for the rain to begin. Sam is still doing battle with the heater, then he has to fix the micro switch in the tap again and that is the morning spent. Between afternoon showers we decide to walk into Monte Carlo to return the usual bag of empties - one day we might remember that the shops don't reopen until 4pm. Hiding the bag of bottles in a bush, we continue through THAT tunnel, and eventually find a good supermarket for all provisions. The 1.5 miles back seem endless, "Are all those potatoes really necessary?" On our return, we retrieve the bottles from the bushes and yield 4 francs on return… every little helps.

October 19th

We are cowards, flinching at the words *pleut, vent, mer, agite* and *orage* in the weather forecast, so pay the 92 francs for another night. Well it did look choppy with a head wind, and we are supposed to be enjoying ourselves! The idea is to take the train to Eze sur Mer and see if we can get up to Eze village, the one we had seen on the hilltop, without going to Nice first as we had been told. We give up – too complicated. As we walk back it rains again and we forget Sam's beers – another day of non events.

October 20th Cap d' Ail to Menton

Time to move on. We escape through the blue patch between two banks of black clouds and think there is a favourable breeze but, clear of the marina, it blows in every direction in turn. Eventually it settles, giving a pleasant six mile sail up to Menton. First, we look in at the old harbour but this appears very full and exposed. One mile further along is the new Garavan marina, where courteous staff are ready to guide us into good position, i.e. opposite the yacht club bar with the toilets and douches next door. The fees are half as much as Cap d' Ail, but you can only book one night at a time.

Each harbour is different, and exciting to us, even though only a few miles apart so no time is wasted before cycling into town to explore. Here are quaint narrow streets with chic, tasteful shops and an ornate Moorish style covered market. Pushing the bikes up and up more flower-decked alleys, we gasp to a halt at a large cemetery. The rows of marble sentry box tombs contain photographs and mementos of the departed. One very ornate tomb is for a Russian Prince, one for Sir Walter Scott and a surprising number of English people. William Webb Ellis, of rugby fame, we failed to find. On the way down, we take a brief look inside St Michael's church, dated 1619. This seems to be more like a theatre than a church. Red and gold damask hangings are draped from side to side and wound around the columns, giving a very dramatic effect, which is said to be left over from the wedding of Honorè 3rd in 1757. I think it will have a few moth holes in it by now! Further down, another Lycra'd crowd of marathon runners surrounds us and the junior Karate Club is enthusiastically kicking out in the square. This is a lively, enjoyable town - but then the Calor gas runs out in the middle of cooking supper.

October 21st

A lazy Sunday spent swimming, lying on the beach, and watching people with their dogs. How do they manage to resemble each other so aptly? I remind myself to become more observant.

Dog rose

25

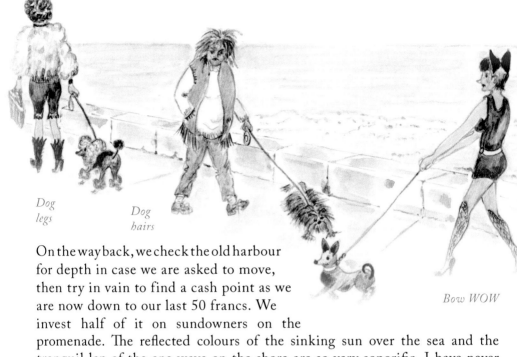

Dog legs

Dog hairs

Bow WOW

On the way back, we check the old harbour for depth in case we are asked to move, then try in vain to find a cash point as we are now down to our last 50 francs. We invest half of it on sundowners on the promenade. The reflected colours of the sinking sun over the sea and the tranquil lap of the one wave on the shore are so very soporific. I have never sampled Pastis before. How is it, that when you find a place where you could be comfortable and enjoy, there is no room in the marina, and why does my bicycle snake its way back to the boat?

October 22nd

Raining again! Weather forecast diabolical. Force 9 wind expected from E/SE, rough sea with dangerous swell later. We prepare to do battle with the *Capitaine* for a further night and find a different man on duty so boldly ask for three more night's stay whilst we have the opportunity. He is concentrating so hard on his computer that we could have asked for a month!

A welcome packet of letters is collected from *Poste Restante* in Monte Carlo. The train journey is scenic and easy, we just chain the bikes to the railings at the station and, surprisingly, they are still intact on our return. Another letter is picked up from the Menton post office, which has a marble floor and vivid green easy chairs. I can't imagine their chances of survival in some of our towns!

The wind only reaches force 8 but it is still enough to make all boats roll, tug and snatch at their lines, and make creaks and groans in harmony with the howling wind.

The next day dawns, it is calm, sunny and warm enough to dry out yesterday's wet clothes. Swimming is not possible though as the swell causes large waves to crash onto the beach making it too difficult to get in. By 4pm it has begun to feel quite chilly and I curse Carl and those wasted three months in La Ciotat.

Heavy rain again, and everyone at home thinks we are having a wonderful time. During a brief lull in the rain, I clank to the shop with the empty bottles and back again with refills and a soggy baguette, to find that Sam has taken out the cooker in order to wire in a gas 'sniffer'. He then disappears down the cockpit locker with an umbrella up for yet another attack on the ailing heater. This ends up on the table again until a slipping fan belt is diagnosed and duly fixed. Count down, blast off! Smoke, more smoke, anticipation. The heater fizzled out again; perhaps we are using the wrong fuel?

October 25ᵗʰ

It is sunny and warm for three hours. The *Capitaine* permits one more night only, then, "You go. You have been here long enough." I think they prefer larger boats that can be charged bigger fees! On cycling to the old port, we are able to book two more nights there instead. We are enjoying Menton too much and are reluctant to leave, but we shall soon be needing a safe mooring for the winter.

The chandlery assures us that Kerdane is the correct fuel for the heater and sells us two bottles so, with high hopes, Sam dismembers it again, finds a broken element to repair … and it still doesn't work!

A little old Frenchman on holiday from Dunkirk, takes great pleasure in telling us that he can wave to our Queen from his window. Well, I think that is what he said!

October 27ᵗʰ

As ordered, we leave. It is only a mile to the old port and the foresail has a much needed airing but we roll like a drunken pig in the heavy swell.

Our allotted space is narrow, and all boats are bobbing and chafing each other. As predicted, the harbour is open and exposed but, it is much more interesting to be near the town centre with its excellent market, and also, it is much cheaper!

There is a Jean Cocteau museum in the old bastion. I am pleased it is free; I think he went to the same school as Picasso. Then there are the Botanical Gardens, with a superb array of vivid flowers, exotic trees and cacti. Sam's observations during this heady meander amount to "Nice hose-pipe!" We also come across the first department store that we have seen and contemplate buying an electric heater, as it is beginning to feel a bit autumnal. There are no douches at the harbour, and it is becoming too chilly to stand under the hose-pipe on the pontoon. A fault in the autopilot has now been mended - we wondered why it sometimes chose to take the boat round in circles.

The day that we should have been leaving dawns black and forbidding with waves breaking high over the harbour wall. I smile at the *Capitaine*, and another 54 francs changes hands.

Rochebrune is an old hilltop village nearby we would like to visit, but that proves to be just too complicated by public transport. After sitting for half an hour in a bus shelter, waiting, plan B is put into action and we set off to cycle into Italy, which is less than two miles along the road. After several minutes pedalling eastwards into an easterly force 6/7 wind, we realise that we had forgotten our passports, so went back for them and started again. The two border guards disinterestedly just waved us through without a pause in their conversation, yet we could have been drug smuggling for all they knew.

It is not easy to appreciate the splendid coastal scenery from inside tunnels, so after the third one we stop, admire the view, ignore the litter, pay our respects to Italian soil behind a bush, then return past the apathetic guards. By now, the sun is shining from a clear blue sky. Should we have sailed today instead of being such wimps, we ask ourselves. The very jagged horizon assures us that we should not. The wind later increases to give a bumpy night, with all warps and fenders making their own weird music.

Reverence

For the next ten days we are beset by the capricious weather and because we are not quite brave enough to face it, we enjoy Menton with its little streets full of surprises. There are so many English people living here that there is an exact replica of an English village church. I decide to attend one rainy Sunday morning, although it is a bit too far to walk in the rain. Parking my bicycle in the porch, I step discreetly out of my wet shorts and into a suitable skirt just as the other worshippers begin to arrive in Burberry macintoshes, tweed jackets, suits and bow ties. They stand dripping umbrellas next to my bike without raising an eyebrow and bid a very courteous, "Good morning."

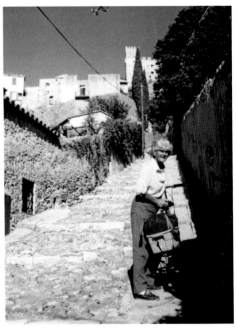

Inside the church, a lady leans over to ask, "Did you lock your bicycle, dear?" (What? Here?)

The service is the familiar *Matins* and it is hard to comprehend that you are not in England – in the 1930s. The main difference is that we all have lashings of red wine in the vestry afterwards instead of tea, and everyone becomes very sociable!

Explorations

There is time to discover more of the charming alleys up flights of steps between tall, narrow houses. Some are dated 1617 and 1649, I try to imagine what the plumbing must be like. Cats lurk in dark corners and you get the

Road to Roquebrune - short cut

impression this is a poor quarter, however it is surprisingly chic and expensive – looking at folk coming in and out of their flower-hung doors.

Boisterous waves continue to pound over the rocks near the bathers braving the heavy surf. I am envious, but it is a bit too lively for us today. What to do on a day when the mistral is still wailing?

One of us has the bright idea to go to San Remo by train in order to enquire in advance about the chance of winter moorings in the marina. What a palaver. We cycle to the railway station, chain the bikes to the railings, then catch a train to Ventimiglia, the Italian border town, which is only six miles away. Then it is, "Everybody out!" First we pass through the Customs Officials and other assorted uniformed staff, then down a subway passing out of the French sector and up again into Italy. There is an hour to wait for another train to go the other six and a half miles to San Remo!

"Whose idea was this then?" we say while we are cashing in £50 worth of francs for a few thousand lire, just to buy coffees and a sandwich. With the exchange rate being roughly 2,000 lire to the pound, it seems like Monopoly money to us! Whilst waiting, we do a necessary crash course in Italian to learn that toilets are called, 'Gabinetti.'

In San Remo, the old port now seems to be owned by the military, thus it is quite a long walk to the marina at Porto Sole where we receive a favourable response for a winter berth. It is not so nice as Menton though. We return to the station in good time, but even the station-master does not know on which of the two platforms the train is due. I think it is meant to be a surprise!

There is the same palaver at the border on return but, glimpses of the boiling sea between tunnels made us glad to be on the train instead of the boat. The harbour master, *El Capitano*, meets us with a request to change berths, he doesn't say why. The wind makes the manoeuvre tricky and we have to forcibly push *Kalivala* in bow to; now we can't get electricity until we buy a different plug! Every port seems to be different.

Distractions

The sea state continues agité, the air is decidedly chilly and, reluctantly, we have to succumb to sweaters, socks, proper shoes and buying that electric heater.

For a few weeks now I have had a loose tooth and tried to ignore it, but now it has flared up and throbs. I know there is a dentist close by as I had chickened-out last week, but now the prospect of it becoming more urgent in Italy, when our vocabulary is still limited to *Dos biere por favour*, *Grazie* and *Gabinetti*, prompts me to make an appointment. The dentist oozes charm and aftershave as he extracts the tooth and 120 francs.

When a Mistral is blowing, the sky is very blue with a few cigar shaped clouds, the visibility is crystal clear and a cold wind hurtles through in angry gusts at regular intervals. The sun is warm, on land it seems a beautiful day but it can last for up to nine days which it does.

During this time, many walks to inspect the sea state are made, and not liking it, we spend much time on a sheltered promenade seat reading and watching the dog walkers and fashions. It is so nice to see little girls in dresses and proper shoes and socks instead of jeans, tracksuits and trainers. The daring creations worn by the more nubile mademoiselles would turn a few heads in our high streets. Sometimes we sit on the rocks, throwing stones into the sea. What mindless occupations for two old would be sailors! At least we don't suffer from stress, that is, not until I run out of Indian tonic.

November 5ᵗʰ Celebration

It is my birthday! The post office with the green armchairs has cards waiting for me. We really must try to do something different today. How about having another attempt at Roquebrune – on the bikes?

Well meaning, but confusing directions send us five miles, nearly all up hill. To cut out the last hairpin bend, we push our steeds a quarter of a mile up steps. A very kindly workman carries mine for the last hundred yards then, unasked, directs us to a bar!

Roquebrune appears to be closed, because it is a Monday. The climb, up countless steps through streets and tunnels, cut into rock are even more incredible than at Menton or Grasse, is rewarded by amazing views across to Monte Carlo and beyond.

Free wheeling the five miles back downhill is painless and exhilarating so we are pleased we made the effort, in spite of much perspiration and a heavily garlicked lunch.

We really must think about moving on – mañana perhaps. Let's fill up the water tank and buy some provisions – just in case.

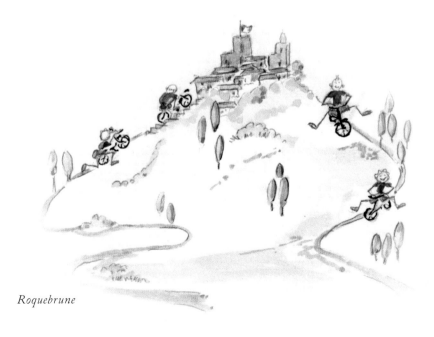

Roquebrune

Chapter 3

Italian seasoning
with sweet and sour titbits
March 11th - July 17th 1991

Relocation

It is typical - the day one decides to leave, there is no wind at all, but there is no swell either so, a disappointment to have to motor-sail the twelve miles to San Remo. The coastline is mountainous yet unpretty, being spoilt by terrace upon terrace of plastic greenhouses. Are they growing tomatoes, flowers or spaghetti?

On arrival, we are guided into berth B67 in this large, new and sterile-looking marina at Portosole. To clear customs and officially enter Italy we must call at the Customs Office. The ensuing activity is like poking a stick into an ant's nest. Much rustling through papers for the correct forms, then for the carbon-paper, head-scratching and, "Anyone got a pen?" The office appears to be run by a team of pimply teenagers in sailor-suits and seem to be quite unconcerned about our yellow flag, (flown when entering another country and free from infection), or what contraband we may have hidden on board.

That done, the marina men, or *ormeggiatores* then come down to change the electricity plug as power is charged extra to the mooring fees, which must be paid a week in advance. We hand over about £80. There is a smart shower block, but being solar powered if you don't dash in at mid-day, the water is *molte fredo* i.e. very cold - as we soon find out! Portosole is now the end of this season's sailing for us. Arrangements are made for hauling out to winter on the hard-standing in the boat yard. Walking round the dockside we meet two Englishmen, Ron has just bought a burnt out 'Gin Palace' to play with, and the other one, Pete, was a naval lieutenant but now is the second mate on a gigantic chrome encrusted, ultra modern motor cruiser. Each of the two tenders on the aft deck are almost the size of our little ketch! He tells us that he has not yet sailed on it, never met the owner who is ridiculously rich but he just has to be ready to leave port at an hour's notice! That does not sound like much fun. Compared with Menton, the San Remo food shops are more down-market and choice is limited. Something must have prompted us to carry our bottles in a box today as the packet of crisps fell straight through the bottom of a feeble paper bag. This is quite a fun place in a run-down kind of way, once you get used to it.

The trains have a comical hoot and the church clocks play a cracked little tune on each face every quarter hour, which is not so amusing if you are still awake at midnight.

Local fashions

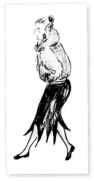

Fur jacket
Black leather
skirt

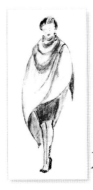

*Purple
Alpaca*

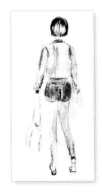

*Brown velvet
jacket & shorts
Brown tights
with pattern*

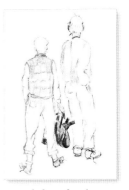

...and then there's us

After a few exploratory outings, we find the 'Bond Street' of San Remo with one shop after another of beautiful designer clothes, shops full of shoes, and leather jackets that have the smell of good leather wafting out through the open doors. All have multi figured prices. We think we are reasonably well dressed in *Timberland* shoes and Yacht Club sweaters but, in this street we feel like two down and outs.

There is a Casino too, but the same rules apply as at Monte Carlo, you must leave your coat. Ah, well, we've been thrown out of better Casinos than this.

November 11ᵗʰ

A pleasant morning passes doing fun things like cleaning cockpit drains and scrubbing decks whilst at the same time listening to the Memorial Service from the Cenotaph in London. I sniffle a bit and we both feel very British.

Behind the marina, across the railway lines, is the promenade and a park, which at some time must have been very attractive, but now is sadly neglected. The trees had been floodlit some years ago. Now all that remains is the broken glass and bare wires. Beyond are grand houses needing lots of care and repair, which are now being used as municipal offices. Much of this town feels as if it has once been splendid and wealthy but its glory has faded, yet it is the principal Italian town from which millions of roses, carnations and mimosas are exported world wide. Perhaps it will be restored in time to come.

Between 6 & 7pm every evening locals like to parade in their finery along the promenade. From the cockpit we can watch and comment on the gold anoraks, fur coats and ultra tight jeans, which make our old denims look passé. Sam is developing a cold!

The Saturday Parade

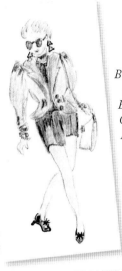

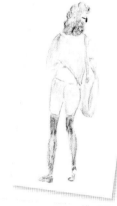

Brilliant magenta
  satin jacket
Black sweater
Gold encrusted wrists
Black worsted
  tailored shorts
Outsize suede bag
Fine black tights
  Black suede court shoes
    with fur pom-pom
    - mink?

Grey tweed jacket
Outsize gold bag
White polo seater
Poured on blue
  sawn-off jeans
Dark brown
  thick tights

Beribboned
  pink hat
Red wool
  sweater
  & skirt

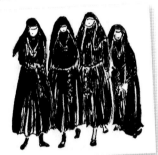

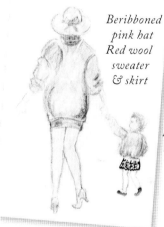

Red jacket
White tights,
  black & check
  dress with
  lace collar

Nuns' chorus

November 13ᵗʰ

There is still no hot water in the showers, the boat shower is dribbly and the last adequately hot shower we had was nearly a month ago, so we now know what a snake must feel like when sloughing its skin!

Trying to book a train and ferry to go home takes three days of hassle. Charmingly disorganised girls send us to and fro between various offices before we finally come to the main office where their computer is down. "Come back in half an hour." Still down. "Come back this afternoon." Still no good. "Come back tomorrow!" The next day, a different girl greets us in a flutter because her computer is down.

Many more quaint streets are discovered in the old town together with a passable supermarket in the main square. Here, we can lock the bikes onto a balustrade to climb up countless steps into more of the older quarters with their squalid alleys, over flowing drains and dilapidated dwellings housing well dressed inhabitants. At the very top, is an elaborate 1630 church, galleried and domed, with brilliant paintings, an altar akin to a marble wedding cake, alabaster pillars and marble balustrades surrounding the shrine of 'Our Lady of the Coast'. All this grandeur seems quite incongruous to the streets that lead up to it.

On the way down in the dusk, we take a few frightening wrong turns, mangy cats lurk in dark doorways then dash out in front of you, there are eyes behind twitching curtains – have we lost our way? At last, in the gloom, we recognise the right path, identified by the pile of dog excrement we had dodged in the centre of a step when on the way up.

After a further half hour wait in the travel agent's, our tickets are delivered from another office and dated 21st November. It is now dark, rush hour and no lights on our bikes! Another scary experience as we play dodgems, down hill on a bumpy road midst the hooting exodus.

The gas bottle runs out again while cooking supper, leaving us with runny eggs and no coffee. Sam is still snuffling.

Now out of range for the Mistral, its Italian counterpart, the Levante hits us. A cold, easterly, force 7 wind is making mischief as we fight with the mizzen and main sails to fold and stow. In the quest to replace the gas bottle, four different shops prove out of stock until 3pm, which leaves plenty of time to browse round the attractively presented chocolate shops, bakeries and delicatessens. Lovely to look at, but with so many noughts in their currency, it all seems madly expensive. How do all these handbag shops and boutiques manage to make a living?

Stopping for a rest at a little bar, the proprietor is very chatty and enjoys telling us how he had run a restaurant in Scotland for thirty years. The taped background music plays *Solo Mio*, not *By yon bonny banks* as expected, but the atmosphere is pleasant and relaxed until we learn the price of two small beers!

Facing the wind now, we walk eastwards seeing more of the has-been fine houses, sad to think of their past dignity. A lane leads down to a stony beach where a barrier of spiked railings offer a short cut back. Warily, we take it.

Gradually, lockers are being cleaned, clothing is sorted whilst Sam potters - he says he is rubbing down an oar. "How do you spell that, dear?"

Two Petes stop to chat. The younger one says he is a crew member on a yacht that has the tallest mast in the world at 165 feet high. This 120ft boat, *Vainquaire* is completely electronic with a television screen in the cockpit monitoring all the instrumentation and the engine room. It is due to leave for Palma, the Azores, then England. We have heard nothing of it since and it will, by now, be quite outdated.

A handsome kingfisher sits on our stern warp as we watch, from the cockpit, the evening fashionistas parade along the promenade. The church clocks multi chime, the trains hoot and mosquitoes grab at our ankles. Shall we be sorry to leave?

The supermarket *Standa* is closed today (because its Monday), so for a few last items, we have to patronise a more expensive one. It is always a relief to get safely back with the shopping when on bicycles, even though we have now strapped plastic boxes onto the panniers instead of trusting the flimsy paper bags provided.

In spite of traffic lights, there seems to be no set system of who has right of way, you just have to be as cheeky as others; it is chaotic. Some Latin men must think they are on a race track.

One hilly road is constructed of the old granite 'sugar lumps', with one in twenty missing. No wonder the beer always has a good head on it. Frequently, we ride the wrong way up a one way street, on the pavement, and through pedestrian areas - we have not been reprimanded yet.

A last visit to the post office yields three letters, before taking another look at posh street in hopes of succumbing to a cashmere sweater. All the wrong colours, and the little woollen jacket for £360 is also resisted.

Everything is now packed, food left overs make an omelette for supper, and as darkness falls black clouds drop down over the mountains, a strong wind howls through, then we realise that we are getting excited about going home tomorrow. Just think, instant hot water, flush toilets, warm house, hot showers and a washing machine!

November 21st

A hot, restless night passes with intermittent mosquito bashing, one finger poised on the canister of repellent waiting for the next fly past. The wind is still gusting hard as we let go of the warps to leave our berth for the shipyard at 9.30am. Sam makes an unusually perfect reverse entry into the lifting bay, only to be sent out again to bump up against the wall until 2pm when *Kalivala* is neatly craned out and put up on chocks to spend the winter

As promised, Ron with the burnt-out cruiser, picks us up to ride in style to the station in his battered, psychedelic Range Rover, for which we are most grateful not to have to carry the baggage for the mile and a half to the train.

After the usual palaver at the border, dragging the bags down steps and up again at Ventimilia, it is a very pleasant journey straight through to Calais, onto the ferry and HOME!

On reflection, much of the weather has not been up to expectation, perhaps it was wrong to set off as late as September or maybe we are losing our bottle. The idea was to see as many places as possible and we have enjoyed the trip despite the lack of sailing.

In seven weeks we have covered 144 sea miles, making an average of two miles per day. Tough going. We have also cycled and walked more than twice that distance. Perhaps next spring we may be braver!

Chapter 4

Hamble to Sanremo

March 11th 1991 Expectation

After four months at home we are looking forward to our return to *Kalivala*. At 10.15am on a damp dismal day we leave, carrying 6 items of luggage, to take a taxi for the train to Dover and a bus to the ferry. It is no disrespect to Sealink that we are taking our own life raft on trolley wheels, plus enough spare parts to build a boat, as well as provisions, two bags of clothing and a few books for ballast! In Calais we transfer to *Wagon Lit* for San Remo, sleeping passively to the rhythm of the wheels until 6.45am, when we lift the blind and are surprised to see that we had travelled overnight into spring. The sun has just risen into a clear blue sky. We are near Arles, passing through the delightful scenery of Provence with fields of fruit trees in pink and white blossom, and primroses along the banks under delicate weeping willows.

As we approach Toulon, Mimosas are in full bloom making the gardens, hedges and embankments aglow with their brilliant yellow. Then comes the sea, living up to its name of Cote d'Azur. What a picturesque journey! Ventamiglia at last, where we have to hump our six pieces of cumbersome luggage down the underpass to the four brass-buttoned, bored customs men, who nod us through with indifference. There was only a ten minute wait for the train to San Remo, a taxi and there is *Kalivala* with a clean bottom, waiting to go back into the water with high hopes of the next few months explorations.

Unfortunately, the workmen had not checked the seacocks and are just going off for a few hours lunch break. If it wasn't for the grinding noises coming from the next boat, it would be quite pleasant sitting high up in the cockpit drinking tea whilst awaiting their return.

At 6pm *Kalivala* is carried back into the water, the engine starts at first turn to motor back to our berth. Now we are ready and eager to be away again to see what delights lie beyond the next headland.

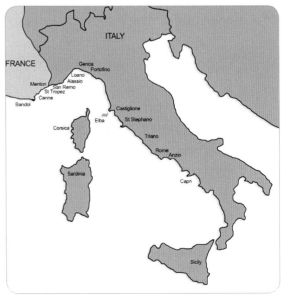

March 12th

Not so fast! There is a number 1 job waiting. After a 3 month rest the toilet has decided not to work. Numerous old spares are reassembled and replaced and that seems to have cured the inconvenience.

The town now seems to be much more awake than when we left, having flowerbeds of multi-coloured Primula along the promenade – and the sun is shining.

San Remo to Alassio

It is a lovely morning to be leaving San Remo. We pay up, return the electricity plug but forget the shower key, so now it has to be posted back. At 9.10am we are out into a hazy, oily, calm sea but with what little breeze there is blowing in circles, it is going to be a boring trip under engine. Within minutes, as we come out of the lee of the bay there is a force four to five head wind, with a sharp chop and white horses spray right over the hood. After putting in numerous tacks and not making any noticeable progress, the gib is furled, and with the motor on we plough head into the waves for 29 miles - and get very wet.

The pilot book said there would be someone there to direct us, but it is not so, and we have some difficulty trying to moor stern – in order to avoid chafing on a large chain on the quay. There is no electricity, but we have a pleasant surprise to learn that the first night is free. A brief cycle ride along the promenade presents an agreeable small resort with a good sandy beach. A force six wind moans through most of the night.

During a further look round next morning while shopping, we come across the famous *Muretto*, a wall that has plaques of many famous people, including Winston Churchill, Gigli, Sophie Loren, Cocteau, many poets, musicians and Max Bygraves!

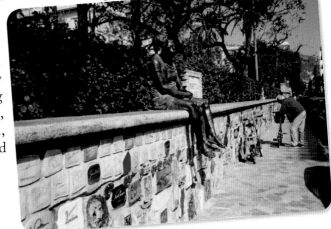

The chance of a sail with the wind behind us prompts our departure at 2.00pm. It is only seven miles to Loana, where we are met and directed to a berth that is really much to big for our 32ft yacht, and we cannot pull up the heavy mooring chain, so have to very quickly improvise by attaching our warps on to the adjacent boats.

At the office we encounter a pimply naval cadet on important manoeuvres (possibly to mop out the toilets) as we pay 14,100 lira mooring fees and 30,000 lira deposit for their electric plug.

March 17th
Clouds. No plans for sailing today, instead Sam disappears down into the cockpit locker yet again, to take out the ailing Wallis heater and fit the new parts that we brought from home. It looks quite promising when a pall of black smoke belches out across my clean washing but, it still does not fire up properly. Next time perhaps.

Later, we walk along the sea front and up into the rather dreary back streets. In contrast, the two churches we find are very ornate with crystal chandeliers and lashings of gold paint, hinting of Christmas decorations. In its heyday, when Loana was a private estate the town hall was a palace.

Although not an inspiring town, we decide to stay another day as we heard there are some notable caves in this region. In the tourist office, a helpful girl with flashing brown eyes gives us maps and bus times. We buy something unrecognisable for lunch, before waiting for the 2.10pm bus, which comes at 2.25pm. It trundles up to the old village of Toirano and on to the caves, which prove to be more interesting than expected.

Italian navy personnel on manoeuvres in Loano Port

There are footprints of Neanderthal man, remains of bears dating back 20,000 years, and countless amazing stalagmite and stalactite formations of alabaster and crystallised aragonite resembling flowers, pillars, draped silk, coral and organ-pipes. The guide speaks mostly Italian in a very soft, reverent manner but throws in a few English words for our benefit, and slips a chunk of alabaster into my hand as a souvenir of Italy. Most enjoyable.

March 19th Loano to Finale Ligure
The electric plug is returned, deposit recouped and dues paid. We pause to look at some new charts but at £16 each we decide to find our own way ahead with the old ones and so leave.

It is warm and hazy with no wind for the first five of the five and a half miles of an unexciting passage to this next plain little town. Its marina has showers and toilets but no power supply, and the bar on the dockside is closed, in fact the whole place seems closed, even after 4pm. The shops are tiny, with a limited choice. At the fifth one, I find a few recognisable items amongst the shelves full of pasta, tinned tomatoes and olives. I cannot recall having bought sausages by the metre before!

The Basilica di San Biagio has the standard ornate frescoes and a boggling excess of decoration.

March 20th Finale Ligure to Varazze

Last night's moorings were free, which compensates slightly for the lack of electricity and local appeal.

'There are clouds' and 'The wind is from the wrong direction' are our excuses for today's lack of enthusiasm, but, another day here? No! Yesterday, the wind changed direction in the afternoon, so on that observation we dare to leave and of course today, the wind stays on the nose with an uncomfortable swell for 15 miles into Varazze.

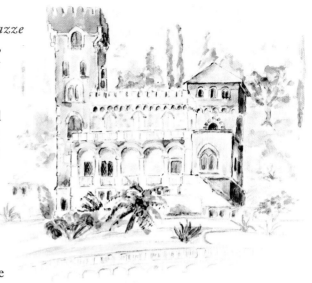

Villa overlooking the Varazze Marina

This harbour looks much the same as the last three places. The offhand *Capitano* does not care where we moor, and there is no electricity again. We must soon get to a proper marina with electricity, as the fridge is warming up and we have already had home-made cream cheese twice. Reading matter is almost depleted and we have not had a newspaper for two weeks. World Radio and Radio Monaco keeps us in touch with news and other snippets, such as an interviewer asking, "Have you any pet hates?"

"Oh, no. I like all animals."

And a customer asks, "Please, do you have any condolence cards?"

Shop assistant: "Sorry dear, we don't do games!"

Varazze

March 21st Depression

From the moment we woke, there was a feeling that today is not going to be one of our best days. The boats are dancing crazily in the harbour, accompanied by the screaming wind and sheeting drizzle, obscuring the mountain tops. We try to remind ourselves that we are here for pleasure as we batten down and look for something to do.

No electricity, therefore no heater. The gas must be getting low, so we daren't use that. Then Sam declares that he is getting too old for this lark and is not sure that he still likes sailing and does not want to go to Corsica or Sardinia or on any long passages. The biorhythms must be a bit low! And I am not too pleased either. In the rain, we try to locate a gas shop and are sent three times by three different, helpful people to the same shop which is full of cylinders but no Gaz. At least we find a modest Co-op on the way. Communication home is not easy;

our phone cards do not seem to work and we have stopped using Poste Restante system since we don't know where we are going next.

When we do manage to ring my son, via Genoa radio on the VHF radio this evening, we learn that my elderly uncle is in hospital with a chest infection and is in low spirits. He is also asking why his nearest relative is gadding about enjoying herself in Italy. I am now suffering an outsize conscience as well as being wet, cold and miserable in a forlorn harbour with a floating dead cat in it. A further phone call to my uncle's neighbour assures us he is not that ill, just feeling a bit sorry for himself and there is no need to return home. There is nothing more we can do but curl up with a book, blanket and hot water bottle and listen to the howling wind.

For the next five days we are storm-bound, with continuing gale warnings. The sea bashes over the 20ft sea wall, the boats bounce restlessly, yet the dead cat has not moved very far in spite of the turbulence. I think it comes in and out with the tide! Sam meets a friendly English speaking chap who takes him by car to forage for Gaz, with some success, but they have to return at 4pm to have our small cylinder re-filled from a large one.

Standing by a door which advertises an English teacher, the lady herself comes along and introduces herself as Patricia from Essex. She is delighted to have someone to talk to and shows us upstairs to her 'school', where we are given newspapers, magazines and paperback books, a bottle of homemade wine and an invitation to use her telephone. Later in the evening we meet her with her nine year old son for a pizza, which makes a pleasant diversion from the pitching boat.

Between gaps in the rain there is a chance to look round Varazze. We are surprised to see irises, stocks and alissium all growing wild on the cliff near the *Lungamare European*. This is a promenade, created from an old single track railway line, which the locals are so proud of that they spend much time strolling along it. One group of oldies starts to spontaneously to sing, led by an 80 year old tenor. We enjoy renderings of popular Neapolitan songs whilst we sit listening and watching the sea breaking on the rocks. Intrepid surfers catch the occasional wave between the rocks scattering the bedraggled pigeons.

On Saturday the town has its weekly market - very lively and colourful with flowers, fruit and vegetables, the usual leather belts and an old lady plaiting palm leaves into a cross ready for Palm Sunday. We buy some soily potatoes from a jolly little man who knows the phrase, "Don't mention eet", as we thank him. Patricia calls with her son Louis and we donate our old paperbacks and magazines to her. Being constrained by the weather has its plus side, you do have time to talk to people and mingle. Spirits are a little higher now, but the dead cat is still drifting around with the surge.

March 27th Varazze to Arenzano
Wow. The sun is shining! Today we will leave Varazze and its dead cat. We wait in vain for the *Capitano* to pay him, whilst his telephone rings incessantly.

A man with a wheel barrow and shovel is consulted, and we think he tells us that the *Capitano* is in town at a meeting, or perhaps breakfast. After hanging around a little longer, reluctantly we do the dishonourable thing and leave without paying for the last few days. Sorry! Five and a half floppy miles in a head wind bring us to Arenzano. We are aware of the sandbar at the entrance, but are not prepared for the rusty dredger at work, blocking the entrance and leaving just a bare boat width between the harbour wall and the plastic cans serving as buoyage. We could have shaken hands with the grinning crew as we inch our way past. The surge of the swell and the beckoning local fishermen on the wall help us into the harbour and show us a space. We have electricity!

Cycling into town to look for the supermarket, we find the municipal park and offices which, the same as Loana, were once a palace (in 1522) and its grounds. All is quite neglected but quite charming with terraces, lovely Cedar trees, Camellias, Wisteria dripping from balustrades, a duck pond and peacocks in full display; not the usual type of council offices! Inside, are richly decorated ceilings, heavy, intricately carved doors and mosaic floors. We thought this should have been worth a mention in the tourist office, but we could not find any history of it.

Whilst we are out, little did we know that the swell is chewing away our warps with the constant tugging and snatching. After an extra hard tug the fairlead holding the warps snaps. We modify with a piece of old chain, and within minutes that also breaks. Next, we try lengthening the warp and that leaves me stranded on the dock. I go to ask the *Capitano* for a quieter berth. He shrugs and says anywhere!

We move, and now we are rocking side to side instead of up and down! It is quite amusing to watch the antics of two electricians fixing the bow lights on the next boat. They cannot understand why the port light comes on at the starboard side and vice versa. After half an hour we feel, we must really tell them that they have screwed them on the wrong side.

Aranzano

March 28th Altercation

Sun, a few clouds – we should have sailed with the light favourable breeze, but we don't. After festooning the guard rails with fresh washing, we walk along to the real port officer, (he has a gold braided cap) to obtain the *Constituto*, which allows us to sail in Italian waters and should have been attended to at San Remo in November.

In the overly ornate church, built in 1751, a young priest told us that the huge dome had been damaged in World War 1 and had been rebuilt and repainted from photographs.

On our return, a force six wind is blowing from the opposite direction and I nearly blow overboard trying to rescue the sheets and towels.

March 29th

Perhaps it was the bump on his head yesterday that affected Sam this morning, but once more, here we go: "I'm fed up with this weather." "I'm too old for this hassle." There followed a short spate of incompatibility due to these defeatist words. "I'm going to sell the boat and go home." "And if you do," I reply, "I would run away because I'm not ready for a life of domesticity, coffee mornings and boredom. And what about seeing Pisa and Rome? We've only come 64 miles since we returned, and that is less than three weeks ago. Wimp!"

After half an hour of silence you could cut with a knife, peace is restored and we enjoy a walk observing more interesting buildings in disrepair; it could be such a nice town if they would mend it.

Sometime in the future, though, it is going to be over run with feral cats, dozens of them and nearly all in kit.

March 30th Aranzano to Genoa

Yesterday's depression is forgotten, today looks promising in spite of a cold north easterly wind. The broken fairlead is replaced, fees paid, and at 9.45am we are edging out of the narrow passage with just a few inches of water under the keel. For once, conditions are perfect enough to give a good sail on the twelve and a half mile passage to Genoa. On seeing the 'Yacht Club Italiano' in the old harbour, we thought it might be more convivial than the Abruzzi Marina. The *Commando* makes us most welcome and insists that we be his guests for the next three days, (Easter weekend), which is graciously accepted. There are lovely hot showers, shampoo, soap, monogrammed towels and a hair dresser – luxury. Perhaps he doesn't have many visitors! We didn't realise that it needs a three-quarters of a mile walk through the scaffolding and plastic curtaining to reach the town. There are glimpses of beautiful old buildings, a cathedral, church and the city gates.

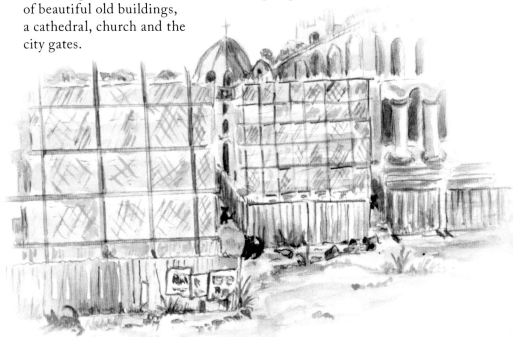

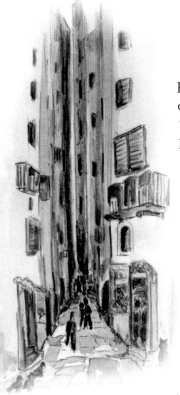

The church is another extravaganza of marble, Rubens' paintings and gold cherubs. Darkened by the eight storied tenements with washing hanging over the tiny balconies, the narrow thronging streets are punctuated with pools of light from small shops aglow with colour. In the litter strewn shadows the stray cats lurk to harass the desultory pigeons. Watched over by muzzled Alsations, wine wizened old men sit in gloomy doorways. It is not comfortable to be a stranger here.

Ode to Genoa

The dead fish float, bloated in the harbour scum
Choked by man's fetid waste, stinging the eyes,
blurring the dazzle of pansy and geranium.
But here at the yacht club see bygone elegance in disguise.

Feathers dragging, care-worn pigeons limp the
cathedral steps.
Lime-splattering the marble to patternless smears.
Now behold the guilded cherubs, saints and painted martyrs
gazing sightless through the crystal chandeliers.

Down the sunless, skyless, crumbling streets,
damp and litter-strewn, where cats slink stealing.
There the shop windows full glow with fruits and cheeses
outshine the dingy walls, damp and grey peeling.

Graffiti on hoarding, boarding and scaffold
hide the sad shame of neglect and decay.
Then glimpse beyond to the proud domes and towers
held high to the sky in praise of yesterday.

All these people, strollers, roller-skaters thronging
the pavements where dark vendors spread their wares.
Do they care? Have they time for thoughts of pity
to save the fate of their noble city?

Genoa has since had much restoration

March 31ˢᵗ

It is Easter Sunday. We think about the daffodils at home and our family, but now there are chores to be done. The wavering windscreen wipers and wobbly king post are tightened up, and some Velcro re-glued that had come adrift from the mosquito netting over the aft hatch. Then there is always some laundry awaiting attention.

By afternoon we are ready to pedal into the so called modern side of town where the local lads pastime seems to be kicking a ball round a large, empty area of concrete car park, or roller skating, whilst the adults are just parading in their finery.

The gardens on the promenade overlook a large funnel-like construction which issues a roaring sound that could more than possibly be a sewage macerator extending concreted coated pipes out to the sea. This is also used for parading on. The surrounding rocks are being used for doing everything else on, including sun-bathing, singing and serious snogging.

The newest section of this area is crowded with strollers over its shiny, patterned tile floor where the North African vendors optimistically spread out their sun glasses, watches and belts. We never saw anyone make a purchase.

There seems to be a lack of chic, as seen in Menton, even the gardens appear neglected. It is rather sad as Genoa has been a very fine and important city in the past. In the 16th century it was raided by Andrea Dorea and has been destroyed and rebuilt many times since. Indeed it looks as if it is being rebuilt at present.

Christopher Columbus and Garibaldi also made their impression here. It is not picturesque, but we are glad we came, even if is just for the free moorings and the very amiable *Commando* who took Sam by car to fetch some oil for the engine. Perhaps we   might return one day to see a fine regenerated city.

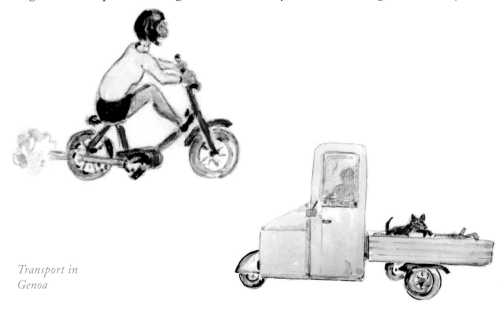

*Transport in
Genoa*

April 2nd Genoa to Portofino

I said we should have left yesterday! There is not a puff of wind for the fifteen-mile passage to Portofino. Once past the urban sprawl of Genoa, the cliffs become steep and rocky with attractive inlets and tiny villages nestled inside. We find the last space on the wall inside the sheltered harbour, in good time for lunch.

This looks better! Brightly painted houses reflect their many colours in the calm waters of this small, quaint, popular town with its lively water-front stalls and bars.

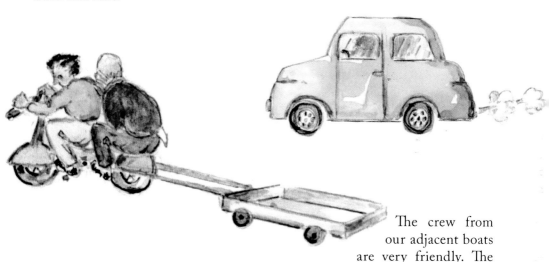

The crew from our adjacent boats are very friendly. The Italian borrows one of our electric sockets and repays with a bowl of pasta, then the French boys invite us to join them for aperitifs and onion bread. Later, we all indulge in a brandy and animated, multi lingual banter.

This is the most socially pleasant day we have spent in Italy so far, even if the sun did disappear over the hilltop at 5pm and Sam had to buy a plug for yet another different electrical system!

April 3rd Portofino to St Margherita

Next morning, after the *Capitano* charges us £10 for mooring and bangs lots of rubber stamps on our *Constituto*, we climb the 200 steps to Castle Brown.

Castle Brown is a fortress dating back to 1000AD, which in 1870 became the private residence of Mr Yeats-Brown, the British Consul in Genoa. It then became the home of the Baber family until 1961 when it was handed over to the Italian Republic. It must have been a formidable home, lightened only by its breath taking views.

Further along the path, passing pretty cliff-side villas, we are surprised to reach a lighthouse on the headland and even more unexpected, an ice cream shop next to it. Between licks, a decision is made to move on. Although it is nice here, perhaps a bit touristy, but what is round the next corner?

No wind again. It does not take long to motor round the corner to Santa

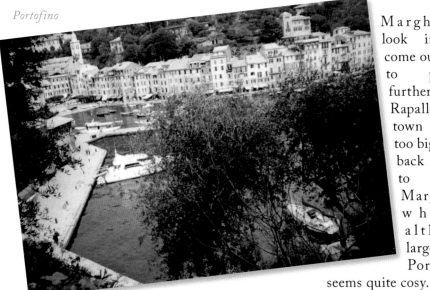
Portofino

Margherita, look in and come out again to proceed further on to Rapallo. This town looks too big, so we back track to Santa Margherita which, although larger than Portofino, seems quite cosy.

After conflicting instructions in broken English and Italian, we tie up and then find that none of our plugs fit the electrics in this port. There are however, adequate shops for all sorts of provisions in the town.

We take a short walk passing several lovely old buildings, which at one time may have been palaces, but now as a sign of the times, have name plates for at least four apartments. One very grand house is bordered by almost a quarter of a mile of six-foot high gleaming steel railings, where a timid little white, be-ribboned poodle sits guarding the electronic gates leading into the extensive, manicured grounds. *ATTENTI IL CANNI* (Beware of the dog), the notice says. Perhaps the Rottweiler is hiding round the corner!

In contrast, the beach is littered with rubbish and the bathing stations are falling apart between the upturned boats where the fishermen sit and chat. On the promenade, vivid flower beds alternate with the statues. Garibaldi is pointing one way, Christopher Columbus points the opposite way, while Santa Margherita points to heaven, or is it another known gesture? Quo vadis!

April 5th

Any plans of leaving today are quickly cancelled due to high wind, heavy rain and a powerful thunderstorm that grumbles on until late afternoon.

Having spent much of the day reading, sewing and huddled in a blanket hugging the kettle for warmth, we venture out at 4pm to look for the official *Capitaneria di porto*, to ask for a weather report. It seems such a simple request but we were not aware that it would cause such a commotion with little sailor boys in a frenzy of activity, running to and fro, jamming each other in doorways and scratching their heads. It is like poking a stick into an ant's nest! They duly return with a telephone number and imply, 'Do it yourself'.

In this place, there are so many uniformed fellows about that you are not sure whether they are high ranking naval officers or car park attendants; they all have a liking for gold braid and brass buttons.

We have never been sea sick but after two days confined below, rocking up against a wall, you get a hint of what it must feel like so – have another gin and tonic!

In our bunks, the body rocks one way and your innards slop the other, and the overhead security arc lamps shine straight through the hatch. It is not easy to sleep when floodlit; battery hens have our sympathy!

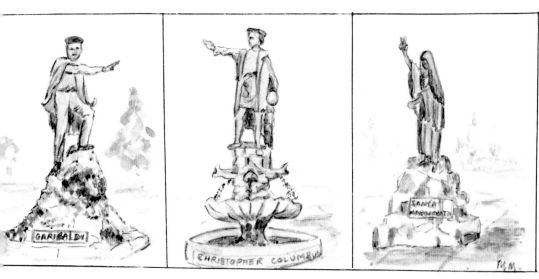

He went this way   *No, that way*   *You're both wrong*

April 6th Lavagna via Sestri Levanti

On leaving one harbour to the next, there is always excitement mixed with some apprehension as to what conditions will be found, ever hopeful that it will be perfect.

In spite of the strong wind, which was forecast the eight mile passage to Sestri Levante is made pleasurable by an escort of dolphins leaping and diving in the bow wave. The town hall looks interesting, but there is very little mooring space. As we make an attempt at a narrow slot, a gust of wind rushes in on cue during manoeuvres to avoid a fishing boat with protruding davits and a floating warp the size of an elephant's trunk. For a few nasty moments, I try to free our bow from under the davits while Sam pokes the elephant's trunk away from the propeller.

We duly escape and reluctantly back track the four miles into Lavagna to the huge, expensive new marina that we were trying to avoid. It proves to be better than described in the pilot book with good facilities and modern shops. The town is lively, has clean streets and a good vegetable market, but one night will be enough since the railway line runs alongside with a very frequent service heralded by an impertinent hooter.

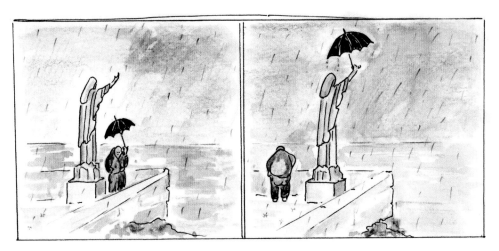

Santa Margherita

April 7th Lavagna to Portovenere
Before leaving this morning some local entertainment is provided by the large boat transporter. Somehow, it has become stuck obliquely on the railway crossing with its load of a gleaming new 36ft yacht just a few inches from the overhead electricity lines! What appears to be the whole population of Lavagna and its emergency services are in full animated attendance, orchestrated by the police and their sirens. A large crane duly arrives and the predicament is gingerly resolved whilst being accompanied by gasps, groans and finally, loud cheers from the spectators.

We dodge across the track between the head scratching officials and back to the boat.

As usual, the only wind is a head wind, but the coastline is interesting with high, rocky cliffs which are terraced for vines, and with little villages tucked into the valleys.

The entrance we need for Portovenere is obscure and very narrow with waves breaking on both sides making us hesitant on approach, until a boat emerges from what appears to be a solid cliff face. Once inside, there is just one vacant space against the wall and the little town looks pleasing.

After five hours of motoring the twenty eight miles from Lavagna, a walk is welcome.

There are 13th century fortifications on the promontory and also Byron's Cave. It is said that he swam from there, nine miles across to Lerici which so impressed the locals that they mounted a plaque in commemoration! The town is bristling with tourists and pleasure boats but yet maintains its attraction - even the church bells sound quaint.

April 8th

Ohhhhh! The bells, the bells! When you have counted the cracked chimes each quarter hour on two church clocks until 3am, one becomes immune to sound and more aware of the rocking caused by the wash from the early fishing boats.

Despite a restless night, we make the climb up a few hundred steps to the 1225 church of St Larenzo, which was sacked then rebuilt in 1460. It has a stark and gloomy air, in sharp contrast to the usual ornate décor. Nearby, the extensive remains of the 1145 castle grimly overlook the little town.

The plan to move on fades when apathy takes hold whilst basking in the cockpit in the welcome warmth of the sun. I am trying to paint when the noise of engines and shouting diverts me. Suddenly, the harbour is filled with activity involving a naval officer and his minions, a police boat, a coast guard launch and two Guardia di Finanza (Customs officials) boats' all chasing a small motor boat; is it stolen, carrying drugs or just part of a James Bond film being made? We never did find out as this was closely followed by a very ferocious dog fight leading to a loud verbal exchange and fight between their owners ... quite an exciting half hour.

April 9th Portovenere to Spezia and Lerici

At last, the weather seems to be settling. It is warm, sunny and clear, but we are twitchy because we now do not have a good up to date chart. So far, we have eye balled our way with the aid of a 1985 Reed's Almanac, a 1982 Pilot book, a road map and leaflets from the tourist offices, and since we have only made short passages close in-shore, it has not seemed too important. Perhaps we might find one in the new marina at Spezia. It is only four and a half miles, and as we turn to go in, three men in a boat zoom up to us waving their arms shouting,

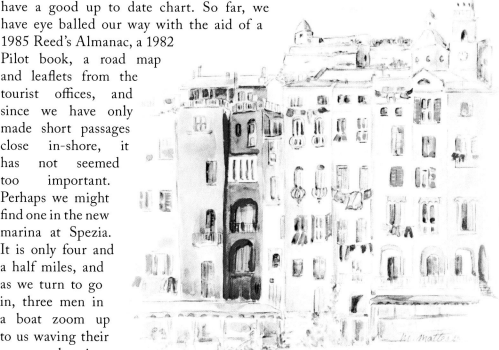

Portovenere

"No room, no room." This does not look strictly true but, not having the vocabulary for cajolement or argument, we try another section. This proves to be private and we can't get out of the gate after finding a vacant berth. Over a cup of coffee, we decide to go the further few miles along the coast to Lerici, which is small and we have no information about it at all.

On arrival, the only available space without having to anchor amidst the fishing boats, is on the fuel dock behind a British yacht, *Red Wings of Troon*.

It is always a pleasure to speak with fellow cruisers in your own language. We learn that the young couple are preparing to cross the Atlantic within the next few days and offer to let us raft alongside them if the fuel-pump attendant becomes peevish with our presence. Three of their out dated, unused charts are bartered for several paperback novels, an American courtesy flag, a spare Q flag, and a glass or two of wine. So now we have charts! The only night noises here are the cooing of the pigeons as they come back to roost in the holes in the castle walls above us.

The fuel man does not return, so we sneak another free night. First, a bit of domesticity. I thought it was time to air the bedding, unfortunately it coincided with Sam's water-play up on deck, resulting in wet pillows and mattresses and a few choice words.

Wherever we go, it always seems to be compulsory to view the church and the castle, which are always up endless steps. It must have kept the menfolk very fit and well occupied hauling lumps of stone up to the highest point of each town in the 11th and 12th centuries. There is a tunnel under the castle which opens up onto three small, sheltered, shingle coves dotted with sun-worshippers and two hardy swimmers. Too cold for us yet.

Kalivala on fuel dock, Lerici

The late afternoon sees a mangy assembly of feral cats mustering on the dock-sides to greet the returning fishermen, strollers licking ice-creams and ourselves sharing the rare treat of an English newspaper, albeit yesterday's. Lerici was also popular with the poets Shelley, Byron and Dante, which is not surprising. How is it that when you find a place you like, there is no space to stay? The young ones from *Redwings* join us for supper and are very happy with our further donation of, *How to cook your catch*, a book of American fish recipes. I'm quite sure we shall never need it.

April 12th Lerici to Marina di Carrara

The pigeons emerge from their holes in the castle walls and a little bird sings in a pink blossomed tree - all most agreeable but, three days on a fuel dock pretending to be waiting for fuel is perhaps long enough before we are thrown out.

First though, we cycle along the promenade, past the Shelley Hotel and the Byron Hotel to telephone the family and check on uncle. All is well.

There is very little breeze until the last of the nine miles to our next stop, but what a contrast in scenery. After passing Punto Corvo, the coastline flattens out for the estuary of Bocca Magra with the mountains further beyond. I count sixteen yellow industrial cranes through a haze of white dust. This is the port that ships marble out, from the many quarries in this area. For centuries this marble has been used by many famous sculptors, including Michelangelo.

This town is very different to any other we have yet seen, it seems quite new. The pavements and kerb-stones of the wide streets are made of marble, so too are the steps up to the church which has a strikingly modern interior with just more and more marble. It is an interesting contrast to the crumbling medieval villages. The old town of Carrara and its quarries are about five miles away up towards the mountains.

There is no room in the town harbour, but we find a space on a curious construction at the Yacht Club. The *Capitano* at the club says we can stay for two nights without charge so, when the sun catches the flutter of our new Italian flag as it glints through the Vino Rossi before sinking slowly over the yellow cranes, we think that this is not such a bad place after all.

April 13th

This morning we catch the 10.30am bus to the old town of Carrara. This is free, as we were unaware that you have to buy tickets in advance from the tobacconist down the street.

This old Carrara is an unpretty mixture of old and new, but has many fine sculptures. The cathedral is under scaffold and its famous rose window

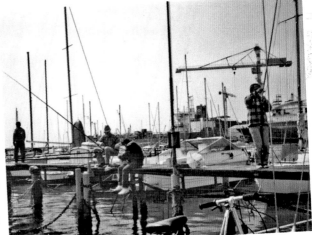

Mooring at Carrara Yacht Club

inside is also being repaired, as is the grand Albertico Piazza.

We fail to find the house where Michelangelo stayed, but come across The Academy of Fine Arts with its balustrades and staircase of gleaming white marble; it is said to be where he learnt his skills. The whole town is obviously geared to this industry and slightly hints of communism.

Bus tickets are honourably purchased for the return which is enlivened by a clamour of noisy schoolchildren.

Marble dust tends to line the throat, so patronising the helpful yacht club bar again seems a diplomatic and therapeutic way to watch the fishermen joking together as they tend their nets.

April 14th Carrara to Viareggio

The wind is blowing our new flag in the right direction, that is until we leave harbour, then it sags limply. The opposite usually occurs when entering.

Leaving the cranes and marble dust haze behind, we thread a way through the many fish-pots and small fishing boats along a featureless stretch of flat sandy beach and distant mountains. For the last five miles there is a welcome breeze, I notice there are a few spiders making an escape when I unfurl the mainsail.

Viareggio is not the cleanest of harbours, but it is well sheltered. We are shown to a berth, helped with the warps and learn that is free. The only drawbacks are that there is no electricity and it is shallow, but four inches of water under the keel should hopefully suffice!

Walking along the canal inlet from the sea, then over a bridge we come to the resort - a bit like the 'Golden Mile' in Blackpool only much longer. There are one after the other of bars, and booths selling pizzas, ice cream and beachwear for as far as the eye can see. The beach is laid out with row upon row of loungers under umbrellas for hire, and the sand is thickly spread with basking bodies and rubbish.

It is yet only April, whatever will it be like in summer?

From the cockpit we can people-watch whilst musing over the giant luxury power boats being built here. Who owns them? Where do they go? Shelley and Garibaldi seem to have frequented this place too!

April 15th

On this warm sunny day we catch the bus to Pisa, roughly ten miles away. The flat, straight road features mainly market gardens, greenhouses (more tomatoes?) and a thickly wooded area. The bus stops close to the city walls, and as you walk through an archway the scene is quite spectacular. First, on one side of the road, you see rows of stalls selling every size and presentation of the Leaning Tower, on tea towels, T-shirts, clocks, purses and hats, together with multiple ice cream, pop corn and pizza stalls. On the other side are wide green lawns, the cathedral, the baptistry and the real Leaning Tower, all built of white, unpolished marble, a truly impressive sight. Unfortunately at this time, the tower is not open to the public as work is in progress to save it from falling over any further.

Designed by Bonnano Pisano, building of the tower began in 1174 and was not finished until some time around 1350. At a height of 186.4 feet, there are eight stories, 207 columns and a deviation of 14.7 feet from the perpendicular.

By the time we had finished our lunch of beer and pizza, sitting on the lawns among all the other sight seers, the tower appears to assume an upright position.

Despite the crowds there is a pleasant atmosphere of peace everywhere we walk, but it is impossible to see all the other fine buildings in one afternoon. Perhaps we might return one day.

April 16th

April 16th

The day begins dull, not conducive to sailing.

"Let's go to Florence on the bus!"

The route is through a broad, flat, fertile valley edged with mountains and miles of lush, colourful market-gardens and nurseries. We pass through Lucca, which is a very old, interesting walled cathedral town, but we have only a brief glimpse of it. At Montecatani, everyone has to change buses onto a rusty old bone-shaker to trundle and bounce the rest of the fifty miles. It is lunch time when we arrive to thread through the narrow streets, picking up a drink and a sandwich on the way to the vast Cathedral Square, which is devoid of any kind of seating. The edge of a flowerpot is shared with two students and a hippie, while the pigeons hang around under your feet waiting for crumbs.

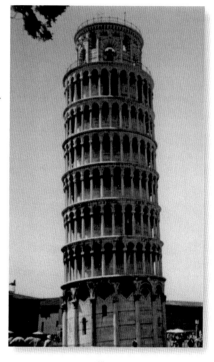

The cathedral and baptistry are not as ornate as some, but it still leaves you in awe and admiration of the sculptors, and the absolute magnificence of the buildings with the golden mosaics and their intricate bronze doors.

The Pitti Palace, Vecchio Palace and Medici Chapel are not given as much time as they deserve, but all have the *wow* factor, although the Pitti Palace gardens seemed a bit neglected, but they must have been splendid in the days of the Medici family.

Weaving our way back to the bus stop through a barrage of market stalls mostly selling leather goods and tatty souvenirs, Sam stops to admire a leather jacket. After beating the price down by several thousand lire, he has second thoughts and leaves a very puzzled stall holder. "It was a good exercise though," remarks Sam. The 5pm bus returns by a much more scenic route through the mountains concluding with another unique sight – a chip shop.

Still being in bargaining mode, Sam now has the cheek to return to the bus office to ask for a 1,600 lire refund on the tickets that we had inadvertently failed to punch on the outward journey. The poor chap is so baffled by Sam's ramblings that he gives in.

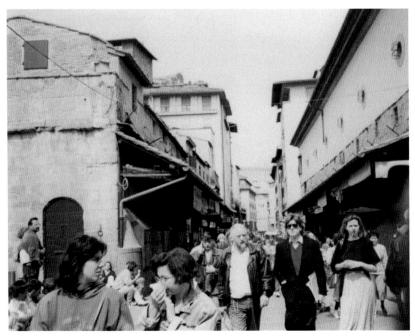

Ponte
Vecchio

A small blot on an enjoyable day is the breaking of a piece off a front tooth just before bedtime, but too tired to grieve about it now.

April 17ᵗʰ
The early morning weather forecast on the radio in English is as follows:

ALL SHEEPSA, ALL SHEEPSA, ALL SHEEPSA. Eastern Mediterranean sea and Nort Tyrrenean sea, wind sout forsa fowr,

There is much rustling of paper and muttering, a pause, then more rustling:

Wind sout estelly forsa siven, wickening. Isolattered toondastorms, sea rowg, scatta-red shoers, modret visibility. ... Bye bye

We do enjoy this disorganised charm! In view of that outlook, and the need of a dentist, sailing is again cancelled for today.

A likeable young lad in an acid green shirt with purple flowers on spends barely ten minutes patching up my tooth for the sum of 50,000 lire, about £25, but well worth it for the amiable, prompt attention, and I suppose some one has to pay for his gleaming, ultra modern surgery.

The rest of the morning is spent following conflicting directions to find a replacement for the gas cylinder and a supermarket. Since we are having to revise our meals to Italian style, it takes much longer when having to try to translate the cooking instructions before buying any thing different.

The barometric pressure falls dramatically and a force six wind blows in, inspiring Sam to take out the Wallis heater yet again and spread out the bits in the cockpit. The fan is checked out - it sounds promising, but still does not work. It is suggested that Mr. Wallis is informed of the appropriate place for his heater.

The predicted 'toonderstorm' sweeps in at tea time, and the radio warns of an oil spillage in the Ligurian sea and mentions Livorno, just where we should be heading tomorrow.

April 18th

It is cold, wet and windy, and we are not going anywhere today, nor, as it happens, for the next four days. Time is passed cutting out Provence material to make table mats, while Sam's project is to remove the fridge motor and mend its broken fan. There is much banging, levering and panting before it relents to being dissected in the cockpit, where it is diagnosed as being more difficult to mend than expected.

The motor occupies the chart-table awaiting inspiration. There is a now a big hole instead of a fridge - just typical that when it is cold, the heater won't work, and when it is hot, the refrigerator is broken.

By mid-afternoon, it is fine enough to trundle the five-gallon can on its trolley to search for petrol for the generator, but we are directed to somewhere way outside of town, so the quest is abandoned. On the way back, catching sight of myself looking like a neglected sheepdog, on impulse, I rush through the first hair salon door I come to and am immediately set upon by a geriatric barber. Twenty minutes later I emerge to the greeting, "Hi, bald eagle," and am more demoralised than ever, having had two traumas in two days.

Back on board, I find the cabin is slowly warming with the aid of the gas rings, candles and hot water bottle before starting on a new, experimental recipe with Gnocchi. The tin of potent bean soup we tried for lunch is becoming audibly gaseous, We are thankful not to have company!

The next day, the weather forecast remains poor. The wind is cold, there is snow on the back mountains, and another thunderstorm anticipated. It is slight consolation to hear that it is snowing in England too!

Dejectedly, we inspect the sea state from the rubbish-strewn, deserted beach and see a very lumpy horizon and the fishing boats wallowing just off-shore. In another part of town, we come across a market - so this is where all the people are, milling round rows of shoe stalls. The whereabouts of the petrol pumps and tourist office have now been pointed out to us.

The remains of the Gnocchi must be eaten tonight, but it is not exactly moreish, perhaps I translated the instructions wrongly.

April 20th Viareggio

More 'toonderstorms' are being forecast; it is cold with fresh snow on the mountains. If we have to stay here longer, we shall need to find out what there is to see in the area. As chicly attired as four layers of boat wear permits, we cycle down the *Golden Mile* to find the tourist office, which is hidden between a pizza bar and an ice cream stall. There are many interesting things to see if you have a car, but the only place within our reach is Puccini's house by a lake five kilometres away, where we plan to visit after lunch.

On our return, we are told that the boat whose space we are in is returning today and we must move, now! The wind arrives on cue just when starting a tricky manoeuvre, but being a little more practised now, we manage to blow squarely into a narrow slot, in reverse, at the first attempt without catching on any chains. It is just my luck that the slimy rope I had to pick up from the wall, splashed a few spots of mud onto a new gleaming Tupperware 'bathtub' in the adjacent berth. I wash it off, apologising profusely under the scowling glare of its proud, muttering owner. He seems also a little peeved that our anchor-lines are effective and his are not so we lend him an extra warp, hose and a deck-brush - and he almost smiles. I think we are friends now! The predicted thunderstorm comes grumbling in, so the trip to Puccini's house is cancelled.

April 21ˢᵗ
Rough sea and cold, but at least the sun is shining, this seems a good day to do the cycle ride. The long straight path through pine woods is a nature park, quite pleasant, but seems to go on forever, not just for five kilometres. Another long road of bars and shops ends abruptly at a lakeside. A small charge of £2 each, admits us into the modest house, which may have been more interesting without the language barrier. The guide speaks no English, but we do understand that everything has been left as it was when Puccini was composing. Here are manuscripts, photographs of the first performance of *Madame Butterfly* in1909, Mimi in *La Boheme*, and letters from Vivaldi and Paganini. One room in the house has been converted into a chapel where he and his family are buried.

After that mental exercise, lunch overlooking the lake is relaxing, before we opt for a different route back. This takes us past rows of bathing stations, bars and booths for a good two miles, then the road suddenly stops and becomes a sandy, rocky track. We follow another cyclist between pine trees and dunes dotted with Azalias, Broom, cacti and sugar cane. Quite pretty, but hard on the knees.

The can for diesel fuel is taken for a walk again later, we find the pumps, but they are all closed and we return in a heavy downpour.

April 22ⁿᵈ Vareggio to Livorno
With struggling sunshine and a favourable forecast, it is time to move on, but firstly, another attempt to fetch fuel and contact the family.

The easiest way to telephone is from a hotel. The staff are quite unfazed when the plastic can, on its wheels, is parked in their rather smart foyer, and they seem to accept the fact that the English are a bit odd. After a visit to the bank, the plastic can now be filled.

With the usual mixture of excitement and apprehension of what the next port will reveal, we leave at 11.20am in a light breeze.

The 22 miles of coastline is flat with dunes and pine forest. A possible stop is in the river Arno at the Marina de Pisa, but this looks uninviting, having fishing nets hanging out into the river on both sides and the pilot book says that the entrance becomes impassable in rough weather. We sail on into Livorno, once known as Leghorn, where the hats were made.

The yacht club official shouts, "No room!" although there appears to be lots of spaces, "Waiting for racing yachts to arrive," so he says! We are to hear that pretext many times.

We circle round looking for a possible space, weaving to and fro to avoid busy tug boats, then warily pick up a slimy line against an even slimier wall amongst a row of assorted, neglected craft.

There is no water point or electricity and all boats are dancing up and down with the wash made by nine fussing, tooting tug boats - but it is free! Entertainment is also free, provided by the activities within the harbour. Several rowing teams at practice noisily dodge between the pilot boats, ferries, and cargo ships that are being pushed into position by the nine bustling tugs.

April 23rd

A force five wind and more '*isolatted toondastorms and rowg sea*' is forecast, which means that we must stay in this dirty corner again today.

The town is busy, has fairly modern streets with an arcade and a department store where we can browse and keep warm out of the rain. In our continuing search for an improved pilot book, we are sent from a book shop to an optician (who also provides weather reports), and he directs us back to the book shop. Everyone is most kind and helpful, but we have no success and there is now a growing need for more details of ports and marinas.

The afternoon jaunt is to look at the Old Fortress and the New Fortress, but we find them both unattractive and so crumbling with neglect that it is hard to tell the difference.

Cycling back, dodging the wrong way down a few one way streets, we come to a high wall between some shops and an office block. In it, are dilapidated doors on rusty hinges, and at the side is a faded plaque which reads, English Cemetery. The doors are locked. "Come back in the morning," says a helpful señor who spends fifteen minutes relating the history of Livorno, Pisa, Florence and the Medici family when he was already late for work.

Further along, is the resort end of town, having a sort of promenade with a fun fair, which is directly in front of the four star Grand Hotel.

The thunderstorm arrives at bed time, just as we are dressing up for bed. The cold nights have brought about a distinct fashion swing; we simply hope that there will be no emergencies!

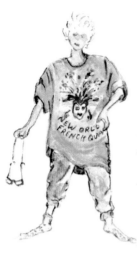

Italian Riviera
1991 Trendy nightware modelled by myself and Sam

Outsize Mardi Gras
T-shirt from 1990 sale
in New Orleans

Pantomime elephant
grey fleecy track suit
trousers with
yellow trim

Off-white wool
socks with
perforated design

Shrunk & faded
1982 Round the
Island 'I'm a
winner T-shirt'

1980 dark red
M&S pyjamas

April 24th

Water and fuel are fetched by the can full to save having to move the boat just to go a hundred yards, then we walk along to the Miseracordia Offices to ask permission to see the English Cemetery. The Señora with the key escorts us to the heavily padlocked doors, and with much rattling of chains, we are allowed inside. What a shock to the senses. The impression is akin to a scene from a horror film. It is quite dark from the canopy of umbrella pine trees, and knee-deep in weeds and brambles. Carefully, we pick a way past the broken urns, collapsed edging stones, debris and wingless angels to read some of the large, ornately carved memorial stones.

Amongst sea captains, archdeacons, lieutenant colonels, and naval commanders are Countess Cowper, Lord Howe-Brown (1822), The Honourable Charlotte Plunket (1816), Lady Stewart, Countess of Mount Cashel, and the Earl of Guildford, all buried between 1700 and 1870. Most graves seemed to belong to someone important. What were they doing in Leghorn we wonder? Apart from a few birds singing, it is hushed, eerie and sad. With a last glance and a slight shiver, we step out of the gloom into the bright, every day bustle feeling as if we have been in a time warp.

Nearby is an excellent market hall, reminiscent of a Victorian railway station, by contrast this has a much more cheerful atmosphere to dispel the gloom of the cemetery.

A bit of boat maintenance involves replacing the ailing water pump with a new one, and now we no longer need to hit it with a stick to turn on the taps.

The VHF radio issues more gale warnings, followed by a very agitated conversation between the captains of two large ships. One captain is convinced that he is on a collision course with the other and is becoming most excitable about it. The other one cannot understand what all the fuss is about since his engines are in reverse as he attempts to anchor almost two miles away right in front of the other boat, we assume. Pity they were not within sight.

April 25ᵗʰ Livorno to Piombino

The day seems fair, so we leave the slimy wall at 7.40am, eating breakfast on the way. Within half an hour on passage, there are high winds and thunderstorms forecast. Hoping to beat them, we sail on under mainsail, mizzen and motor.

Most of the coastline is flat and boring apart from a few dunes which are reputed to be a nature reserve for deer and tortoise, and other parts of the coast are industrial.

The wind pipes up in the afternoon causing a tedious, short choppy sea. The scenery improves near Cap Barratta, but the conditions do not, even so we are tempted to go straight across to the Isle of Elba, then the thought of another two hours on top of the seven we have already done, prompts us to just make for the nearest port, and that is Piombino.

Well! If we thought that Livorno harbour was a dump; see this. Ahead, another yachtsman is searching for a space, but whilst waiting in hopes of rafting alongside of him, a fisherman beckons us over to a long high wall which we assumed was only for big ships. He kindly takes our mooring lines and ties up against a huge commercial fender. Too late we realise that we cannot get ashore, the wall is too high, and after 48 bumpy miles we are trapped in the most unsightly place yet.

There are coal-hoppers bucketing slack, chimneys belching black smoke, brown smoke and steam, gasometers, sheds, and pyramids of coal and rubble. Being now too tired to invent a method of scaling the wall, we sit in the cockpit in a weak hint of sunshine, watching the dust settle on the gin and tonics, and remind ourselves that we are doing this for pleasure, so enjoy it.

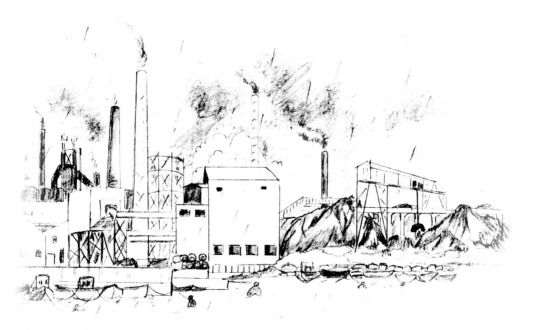

Piombino. Gem of Tyrrhenia, Gateway to the Islands

All night the boat bangs and snatches in 40 knots of wind and driving rain, which Sam bravely faced several times to adjust the lines and groaning fenders.

Daylight reveals *Kalivala's* decks completely covered with a layer of coal dust, grit and debris, which has blown down from the top of the dock – and the folks at home are envious of the wonderful time we are having!

In the rain, somehow Sam manages to climb up and find a hosepipe to join onto ours, so as much grime as possible is flushed off before breakfast.

A sailor boy shouts down to tell us to report to the *Capitano's* office. Yes, but how? Several ways to scale that wall are tried out: the bosun's chair, swinging the boom out and balancing on two boxes, but no way feels safe. Sailor boy drips back with a friend – it seems that the officials are becoming impatient. With limited words and some explicit miming, it at last dawns on them that we are having some difficulty in obeying instructions. After a pause for thought, we put the ship's papers into a plastic bag and pass them up on the end of the extending boat hook. No need for us to get wet!

Just as we are thinking up another means of escape, the *Capitano* himself arrives, all brass buttons and braid, accompanied by his underling. He sizes us up and says that one person must stay on board at all times, which is quite an unnecessary request at present, then satisfied that he has made his presence felt, struts away.

Not to be defeated by this wall, I volunteer to stand on Sam's shoulders near the giant fender, which looks like an old tractor tyre and scramble on to it, then one foot into an iron ring, pull on a warp and I am up on the dock. The view is no better on the mile and a half walk into town but, to compensate is the best supermarket I have seen while being away, so I stock up with as much food as can be uncomfortably carried .

The rain starts again, then help! How do I get down? The boat-hook rescues the bags, and with a slither and a bump I hit the deck.

When sitting below, you can just see the different coloured smoke chuffing up from the chimneys of the iron foundry. The Romans found iron here in 600BC – we wish they hadn't as the decks now have another layer of dust and grit. Again we ask ourselves – are we having fun yet?

April 27th Piombino to Portoferraio, Isle of Elba
The day is murky and uninspiring, but the thought of another day in this mucky hole gives us courage to leave. It takes almost half an hour to unravel all the grimy warps, then away to what had appeared to be a calm sea, but is actually a large swell left by the storm.

Navigating to Portoferraio is simple – just follow the ferries for fifteen miles. Even under a black sky, Elba looks inviting with its picturesque coastline and hills. For the first time, it is necessary here to use our own anchor and then reverse into a slot to tie up stern-to onto the harbour wall. Although being a bit out of practice with this method it works well, except for the few moments when I trap my fingers between the winch and the anchor chain, it is an unforgivable crime and I do know better.

On one side there is a yacht from Cheshire, then shortly an Italian boat arrives at the other side and asks us to come for drinks at 7pm. The first priority though is to scrub the iron foundry out fall off the decks by bucketing up sea water as there is no tap water here unless you pay for it. There is no electricity either, but the mooring is free. After we scrub ourselves, we are ready for the 'party' this proves to be – half a tooth, a mug of white wine and a few peanuts in the company of six wealthy, yet charming Italians, all speaking perfect English... Piombino is soon forgotten.

April 28th – May 13th Portoferraio
The blue sky and sunshine lift our spirits in this pleasant harbour. It is busy with traffic and people, yet it feels safe and an interesting change to be in the midst of the 'stirrings' where passers by stop to chat. A Canadian lady who is out jogging, invites us to their boat which is up at the boat yard, the Italians call to say goodbye as they leave for Marciano, and then I see a little old man standing smiling at me from the dock side. Going over to say hello to him I am greeted warmly with a handshake, two kisses and three boiled sweets.

From our berth we can also be entertained by the happenings at the tall flats across the road. On the fourth floor, a saucy señorita sun bathes, seductively sprawling on her lounger after draping her clothes over it. A lady on the third floor guides her old dad out to a chair on her balcony where a fluffy white cat sits preening beside him. The second floor balcony has washing hanging over the balustrades, and the ground floor doorstep is being vigorously swept.

Without having to look for 'the man with the key', one source of water is to be found at a tap in a remote corner – after dragging the drum through a square and three archways. The locals now tell us that dead dogs and swimming rats have been seen at its source and so it is not recommended for drinking. Too late.

As the sun goes down, the strollers come out. Uniformed callow cadets idle past, eyeing the giggling girls who, in turn eye up the boys. Another cadet strolls by with his arm round a naval officer, two Germans stop and chat, then old dad, up on the balcony, staggers to his feet scattering the cat and relieves himself into the pot of geraniums, which percolates through and down onto the washing on the second floor balcony. It is much more entertaining here than watching television.

Moving further along the coast to Marciano marina is mulled over but, by now we have met several British cruising boats and it is so easy to be able talk and laugh together that we are a bit reluctant to move. Firstly, we will inspect the town by bus. This is a most enjoyable hour long drive over twisting mountain roads, by meadows, a riot of colour with wild flowers and views of a spectacular coastline and vivid blue sea.

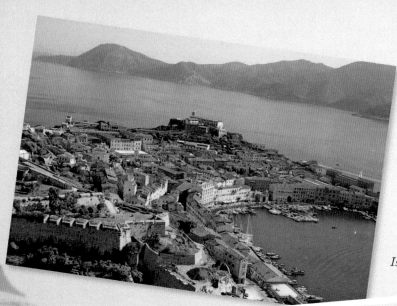

Island of Elba

Napoleon's Villa Martina

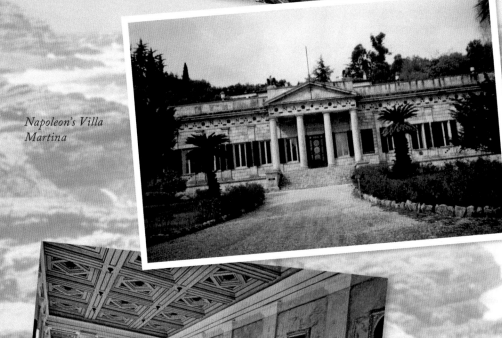

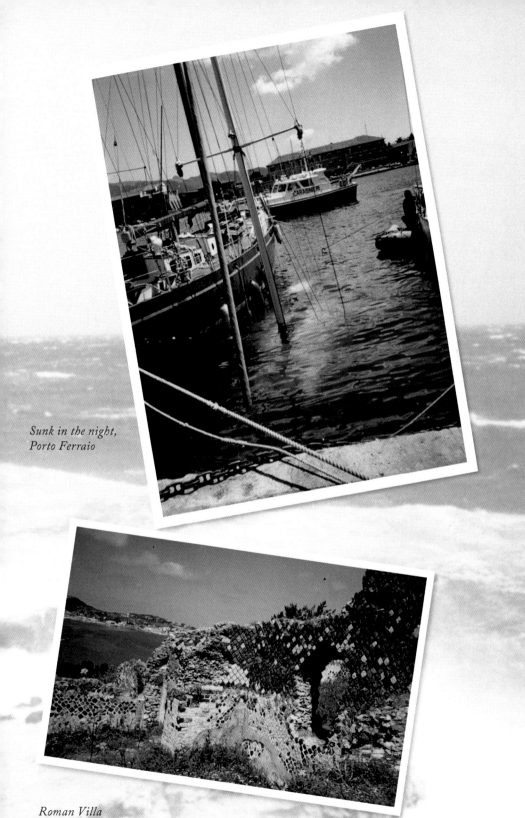

Sunk in the night,
Porto Ferraio

Roman Villa
2ⁿᵈ century, Elba

Marciano is a quaint little town with alleys, archways and a morning market. There are not many yachts here, the depths are dubious. We look for the Italians, but they have already left. Porto Ferraio is certainly more fun!

The 3pm bus back is a battered rusty heap, and the over-eager driver has a few close encounters on the tight corners and has to reverse out of the bushes on a bend when another bus passes too closely. It is quite a relief to safely return to the boat where we spend the evening socialising with yet another new arrival, who invite themselves aboard bearing a ten inch pizza and a pitcher of local brew. Now there are five compatriots in a row. We watch two more boats arrive which seem to be having anchor problems, and just hope that there are not four other anchor-chains over the top of ours.

There is much here yet to be seen. Elba was the home of Napoleon during his exile and his summer residence, Villa Martina is just a few miles out of town, and open to the public. Taking the bus one day we find it is closed and deserted. Next day, using yesterday's unstamped tickets, the scene is very different. Twenty coaches in the car park spew out tourists and bored schoolchildren.

Once inside the villa, there is not much furniture in the tatty, 3D painted rooms of this under whelming building, although it did contain many fine battle paintings and lithographs. In hindsight, we could have saved our entrance fee by just looking through the windows!

Another boat from Jersey arrives in the harbour, and its crew are so delighted to be able to communicate that they serve an admirable gin and tonic.

The hot of press news one morning is about a yacht further along that has mysteriously sunk during the night. It causes much ado with the gold braid and brass button brigade. Not wishing to appear too nosey, we catch the 9.30am bus across the island to Azzuro, which goes via Capolivera, a small mountain top town, then back down through hillside vineyards and meadows to the coast. The town of Azzuro is compact and pleasing, but the harbour we are interested in is very exposed.

Sitting in the square, drinking an over priced, tepid Cappucino, it is agreed that we do not move round to this place either, so we catch the next bus back and enjoy the scenery again.

There is more activity on the dockside at 1.30pm when divers place buoyancy bags into the sunken yacht. Nothing happens quickly here, so it is 3.30pm before a crane arrives and a crowd gathers to wait for two hours to see it slowly rise to the surface where firemen pump it out, and the crowd disperses. It is said that the owner slept the night on a friend's boat, forgetting that he had left his water tank filling. 'Yeah, yeah, yeah. Is it just co-incidence that it is up for sale and the insurance might be useful?'

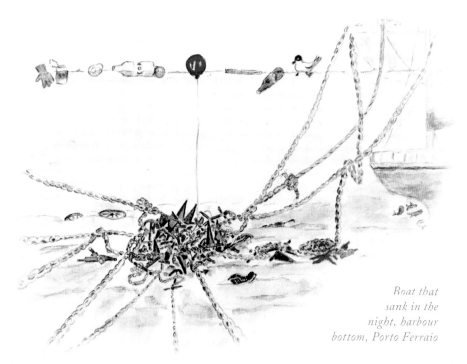

*Boat that
sank in the
night, harbour
bottom, Porto Ferraio*

More relics of Napoleon are found through an inconspicuous doorway up a narrow street of steps. A sour-faced guard issues tickets at 25 pence each to see Napoleon's death mask, a flag, a replica of his coffin and a few bits of memorabilia. During the few minutes of viewing, there has broken such a sharp thunderstorm that the rain is cascading down the steps like a waterfall, whilst down at the bottom, the streets are awash with six inches of fast flowing rivers and the traffic is in chaos.

Taking off our shoes, we wade back to find a Canadian boat moored next to us, and its two crew waste no time before coming across with a two-litre flagon of dubious-looking Corsican wine. To our great pleasure, after exchanging advice on several harbours, we swap our French pilot book for their Italian one.

Our intentions to move on are daily thwarted by the demands on our social calendar, which is taken up for at least another week by all this cruising fraternity with a great need to laugh and understand each other. Hence we have lunch dates, afternoon tea gatherings and supper parties then, we all go to a fish restaurant or for a pizza in the lean-to tarpaulin extension to a shed-like café. Saturday night is safari night, when each crew provides a supper course and you tramp from boat to boat to eat it. As expected, next morning Sam is complaining of acute arthritis – of the head, but of course it can't possibly be the wine to blame! At 10.30am he is stretched out with the Union Jack and a gladiola on his chest, getting no sympathy from me. He comes back to life in good time for a cycle ride up out of town to a promontory, Pte di Grotte, which looks across the bay and to the mountains beyond. Here are the remains of an extensive 2nd century Roman villa carpeted by a vivid array of weeds, yellows, blues, purple and magenta, wild gladioli, vetch and broom pictured against an ultramarine sea. A plan of the villa would be helpful as it has obviously had baths, drainage and heating. The outer walls are of dark granite and pale grey flint mosaic in geometric designs. We see no notice board telling its story, but it is certainly of some worth, as three coach-loads of Germans suddenly disturb the dust with video cameras and 'wonderbars', then drive away again within minutes!

Back on the dock, we learn that a new arrival has reported 50 knots of wind on passage from Corsica and also, that a cruise ship has come in full of frightened farmers from Greece. They have had such a rough crossing that they are now too scared to go home!

We are so thankful that we are not planning to leave just yet, in fact, it would be no hardship if we have to spend all the summer here.

The weather is still fickle, and old dad on the third floor has not been put out to air for several days – he acts as a kind of barometer. Between welcome interruptions from our new friends, the normal chores and some maintenance has to be done. By balancing in the dinghy, Sam is gradually cleaning the oil from the hull that we picked up in Livorno harbour, and the plugs in the teak decking are having to be replaced a few at a time. After staying for coffee, the skipper from the Cheshire boat takes our ailing fridge motor away for checking, but returns it later with a shrug.

Every other day my Italian boy friend comes by, stops, smiles, shakes my hand, puts several sets of kisses on both cheeks, then hands over the three boiled sweets. On Sunday, he is very smart in a suit, having been to church. I think he is lonely.

At a Pimms No1 lunchtime convention, on board the Canadian yacht, one of the members proposes an early supper in order to climb to the top of the fortress to watch the sun set over the sea This is seconded by the Jersey crew and unanimously agreed. Alas, someone's calculations taken from *Reed's Almanac*, are a bit in error and we almost miss it, perhaps he was still on GMT.

It is a very pretty sundown, and we just catch its last glimmer as we all reach the viewpoint gasping for breath. Whilst we are out, yet another yacht has come in, said to belong to a well-known artist who also has his wife, two small daughters and an immense St Bernard dog, which is as scruffy as the boat and barks at all passers by until well into the night.

Each day the artist sets up his easel and his exhibits on the dock in hopes of making his fortune, but we did not like his paintings and I don't think anyone else did either.

I wonder if we should consider moving on? There is a friend wishing to join us in Brindisi on September 6th to help on the passage to Corfu, at this rate of progress we shall not be there in time, but that is too far ahead to worry about now.

May 13ᵗʰ Porto Ferraio to Castiglioni della Pesca

The St Bernard alarm clock goes off before 6am and continues, so perhaps this is a good time to leave. At 8am the anchor comes up with surprising ease, without having become entwined with the other chains. With a little sadness, we wave goodbye to all our new-found friends and reluctantly motor out of the harbour. It has been a lovely holiday, but we are on a mission to Greece and beyond.

The hazy coastline is attractive up towards Azzuro, where Elba is left behind to head back to the mainland, still having to motor, due to a lack of wind. There are two small islands, each with a fortress and much debris of logs and large branches with birds still sitting on them.

After 30 miles, the wind arrives on cue just outside the Castiglioni harbour, blowing confused waves up into its shallow entrance. There is no space near to town, the depth-finder shows 2:2 metres and the alarm starts fussing – ignore it, we only draw 1:5 metres. Now heading for the yacht basin we are at once blown across the anchor-chains with the depth alarm going berserk, still finding no space and almost no room to turn round.

Faced with the alternatives of returning seven miles to Punta Alla marina at a cost of £40 per night, or going a further 20 miles, we opt for hanging fourth boat out on three neglected-looking other craft.

Within a few minutes of setting the lines we hear a shout, "Halloooooh! I'm Janet McDuff, who are you?" She climbs across the boats and after finishing off the last of our wine and crisps, invites us round to meet her Italian boyfriend, Mario on his very traditional 1964, 12m gaffe-rigged schooner. They are both very young, with high hopes of chartering the boat but Mario does not seem happy about his country in many respects. A new law has put a £2,000 tax on the boat and a lesser amount on his motorbike and he cannot pay, so they must either, escape from Italy or put his boat in Janet's name. Either way, he is very upset and in tears. They give us some advice on where and where not to go, but we think they are glad to have someone to listen as they unburden their woes. We feel sad for them, or were they expecting a hand out?

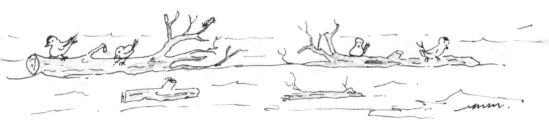

May 14ᵗʰ

The bikes are humped across the three other boats onto the quayside to go and explore the surroundings. The beach area is nice enough, the tourist office is helpful, and there is a useful supermarket. On advice, we ride out into space to find *Casa Rossa* (The Red House). This is a derelict has been, built in 1765 for the Grand Duke Peter of Lorraine and looks like a disused cotton mill. Not being very impressed we return, chain the bikes up outside the old walls and walk through the narrow, pretty streets of the old town. At the top is a shady square, church, fountain, a privately owned castle and lovely views down to the sea. Not such a good view, is a yacht getting stuck on the mud three times when attempting to leave the harbour.

Back to necessities, taking the water can, here again you have to ask for the key to get water. Sam manages to fetch three cans before the very churlish old man demands its return, but later that night, a guilty pair of mole-grips sneak out to acquire a fourth can full, so now thankfully, the water tanks are full.

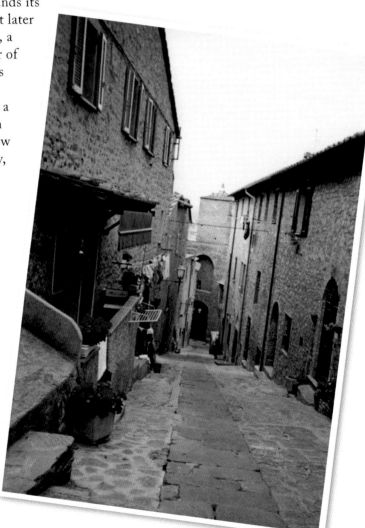

Castiglione old town

May 15th Castiglioni to St Stefano

An early morning mosquito raid wakes us. The day looks fair and we are ready to leave before 7am. There is little room to manoeuvre, barely sufficient depth and the sand-bars at the entrance to nudge past, as we try to recall where that boat went aground yesterday.

"OK. You can breathe out now, and put some sails up!"

Apart from having to avoid a few fishing boats and their nets, it is a pleasant 24 mile passage. It is when you arrive at your destination that the hassle begins. When one man tells us to go into one place and two others say different, then to be shoo'd out of the harbour and sent into the old port, which is just an exposed wall with iron rings in its side. Here, we have to drop anchor and reverse up to the wall between a small yacht and an 80ft gaffe-rigged ketch used as a diving boat, where someone helpfully threaded our warps through the rings. With a long leap, I go along to ask at the marina for a more suitable place where I'm given the same old story. "No room. Regatta on Saturday."

There is no other option but to stay or go on another fifteen miles. It is not really comfortable here but we stay, in spite of the comment in the pilot book that, 'Strong winds from the north render this harbour untenable, and you must leave and anchor in the bay.' Looking up the word untenable in the dictionary, the definition is, *that which cannot be maintained against attack.*

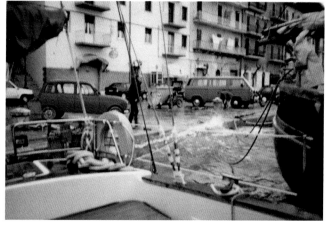

"Oh, well. Let's hope for a calm night. We are too weary to worry about it now, and anyway, the big dive boat might shelter us. It so happens that five Germans need to tramp across our deck to be able to reach the dive boat, where they laugh loudly into their *steiners* until well after midnight.

Untenable

May 16th

Everyone knows about Sod's Law. At 4.30am we are awakened by an appreciable rocking, which at first we take to be caused by the wash from the fishing boats, so try to settle down again. It becomes more uncomfortable and concern for the warps draws us reluctantly out of bed to find the waves bouncing all boats around like corks in the force 6 wind from the dreaded northerly direction, the untenable one.

By 7.30am conditions have worsened, and the large boat we hoped would act as a buffer, is now much closer and soon is pushing against our beam with all fenders whining in protest. The pilot book said we should leave and anchor in the bay, but by now it is obvious that we will not be able to take up the anchor and neither can the *Swedish Halberg Rassy* on the other side, as the big boat's chain is now over the top of ours. Much shouting eventually rouses the night watchman of the dive boat – a drowsy young lad in pyjamas, who gapes at the scene in horror, but does not know what to do about it. After adjusting the fenders, he disappears below. There is no sign of the Germans, they are guests, so sleep on.

At 8.30am we are in the throes of a nasty situation. More fenders are tied on and the warps slackened, but the hulk is pushing very hard and we are going to be slowly crushed, we will surely lose *Kalivala* and there is nothing we can do to avoid it.

We are cold, quiet, and very frightened as there is no way to get ashore now since slackening the lines and we are too far away to jump.

Preparations are made to abandon ship. Into a black plastic bin liner go the ship's papers, passports, wallets, a few items of clean clothing, (don't forget your knickers), a packet of biscuits and I forget what else, it is like a bad dream.

Somehow, the young lad manages to get ashore and fetch two other men who tighten up the anchor chain, which at once, slightly relieves the crushing motion.

In full oilskins, life-jackets and harnesses, we can only stand waiting and watching in the pouring rain, and try to console the Swedish couple on the other side. They are even more afraid than us as they have two young sons with them aged three and five years old.

After what seems an eternity, the boat owner arrives and very skilfully inches it forward to gradually take up more slack on the anchor chain without snagging our chain with his propeller. With still no sight of the Germans, what a relief it is to see him drop anchor out in the bay.

There is now the full blast of the wind on our port side, but the danger of being crushed has gone and there is nothing to do but sit it out and watch the waves washing over the quayside flooding the street.

Two more tense hours pass, and by 11am the wind drops to a force 2, the swell eases and the two little Swedish boys are out on deck happily playing with their fishing nets and toy boats, while their poor father is so scared and ready to give up and go home. We lend him a pilot book!

The lull only lasts until early afternoon, then the storm is back again in full fury making us thankful for the extra warps we put on during the calm. In the late afternoon, when the sun shines, we buy the two little boys an ice cream then sit studying cloud formations, hoping that whichever 'front' it was has now safely passed.

We become quiet and despondent. "So this is idyllic cruising in the Mediterranean?"

"Do we need this sort of hassle? Is it all part of the fun or meant to be character building? Perhaps the adrenalin output may counter balance our cholesterol intake and give us eternal youth." But really all we hope for is a quiet night.

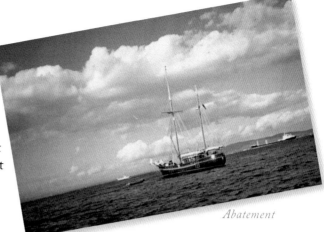

Abatement

May 17th *St Stephano to Cala Galera Marina*

The day seems bright and promising, until we look towards the hills and see the thunder clouds assembling. With only a fourteen mile passage to the next port, we agree to take a chance and hope that we can arrive there ahead of the weather system. A few silent words with a higher deity about the situation ensue, and we just hope that *He* is listening.

The anchor comes up surprisingly easily. A light breeze with a slight swell makes a reasonably enjoyable sail. I cannot remember which of us noticed it first, but in true pantomime fashion the cry is, "Behind you," and we see this gigantic storm system fanning out threateningly, somewhat marring the pleasure of the picturesque coastline as we wonder, "If we are sailing at six knots, at what speed does a storm travel?

As we pass the Isle of Giglio this mass of weather is still making advances, but it could pass sideways and miss us. What we have forgotten is that we are only sailing round to the other side of a large headland, so sure enough, the storm is waiting for us at the fuel dock, having taken a short cut across it. Pow! 30 knots of wind from nowhere hit us. An Olympic leap, with a warp in each hand, much heaving and a trip up over a cleat, we are secure.

A space is allocated but we have to be helped by the very courteous staff in their dinghy, who push and manoeuvre *Kalivala* into a very narrow gap, take our warps and make them off. Next, they lend us the correct plug for electricity and point out that there is both potable and non-potable water for each berth. With all this considerate courtesy in a heavy down pour, you can feel this is going to be expensive. In spite of being on the furthest extremity and nearly half a mile from the office, facilities and shops, it feels like heaven.

When the vicious little storm passes, we cycle into the nearby pleasant small town of Port Ercole to enquire about moorings, but get the usual response from the gold braided shrugging shoulders, "No room for visiting yachts."

We look for Sigfried and his two little boys, wondering if they are here or still banging on the wall at St Stephano, but are soon side tracked by the sight of a good supermarket. The sky is looking menacing again as we pedal back, wobbling with an overload of Italian fare.

Our return to the boat is greeted by shouts and beckonings from some Germans on a nearby boat. They are on top of the high sea wall and becoming very excitable, so we prop up the bikes and scramble up the ladder; and there, just over a mile off shore, descending from a menacing mass of 'cauliflower' clouds is a water spout! Watching through binoculars, we can see the ferocity of this awesome phenomenon as it slowly approaches. The spray of water as it is sucked up into the vortex, is also clearly visible. A brief squall sends everyone for shelter, leaving us thankful that none of us was caught out at sea.

This is a pleasantly situated marina with a good shipyard that has all the facilities for repairs and hauling out, ideal for wintering, and you can even get a print out of the weather forecast – in Italian.

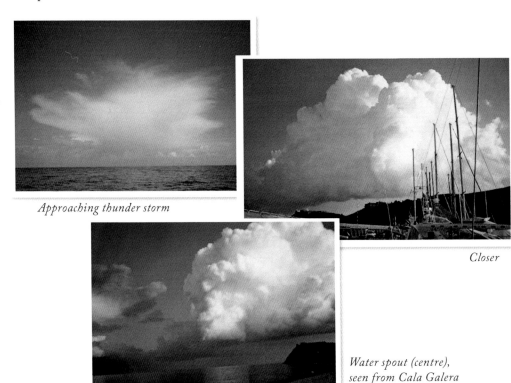

Approaching thunder storm

Closer

*Water spout (centre),
seen from Cala Galera*

May 18th

A warm sunny morning prompts some enthusiastic deck scrubbing. It is now three weeks since we have last had use of a hosepipe to be able to properly fill up the water tanks and finally get rid of the Piombino grime. During that time, we have been very stingy with the washing water, so the next luxury is in the marina showers, which are hot and clean. Oh the bliss! And I can now plug in my hair drier and hot brush and begin to feel human again. It is surprising that all the things we take for granted at home, like switching on lights, taps and kettles, become an appreciated luxury on board.

There is a small supermarket on site, selling *Carr's* water biscuits, Robertson's jams and many other English products at extortionate prices, but I only buy bread, which resembles volcanic rock, yet it is really very good.

At lunch time the wind arrives suddenly from force 0 to a force 6 within seconds, bringing rain. Will it ever settle?

Later, we cycle round the bay, admiring the opulent villas tucked away in manicured gardens, with an occasional Lamborghini or Alpha Romeo parked in the drive just visible through the security gates. Nearby is a sandy beach, a hilltop fortress and, growing wild, Verbena for the vase and Rosemary for the chicken supper.

Now comes more rain, it is quite cold so it is further luxury to plug in an electric heater and switch on all the lights, making sure that we have our money's worth, as £15 per night seems a high price to us in 1991.

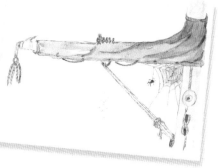

Force 0 wind

May 19th

After a peaceful night, dawns a bright, sunny day. Through the clatter of washing up, we hear a shout, "It's got to be Sam Matterson", and there on the dock side is a chap called Harry who we have known for many years whilst taking the Yachtmaster exams in the heart of the Midlands. Expressions of surprise, pleasure and incredulity follow as we learn that he is on his way to Corfu with his lady and her father, to put his boat *Simetra* on charter. To have the opportunity of English conversation is always welcome, but to meet people you know in the middle of nowhere is quite amazing! However, there is work to be done this morning, so we invite them for tea. Sam continues replacing the teak deck-plugs, whilst I make full use of the abundant hot water in the laundry. On a further attempt to find the entrance to the castle fortress, we learn that it is now a private residence.

Tea time extends into wine time and then supper, while we all catch up on our news and plans. These include thoughts of moving on tomorrow, as we don't wish to afford these prices.

May 20th

We wake early, all psyched up to leave but the sky looks wrong. There are mares' tails fanning out from a solid dark cloud, but no wind. The forecast, due at 9.30am does not happen. All this uncertainty is affecting us, we are becoming very twitchy and a bit cowardly.

Our friend Harry and his crew are ready to go. We say our goodbyes, make a decision to stay, despite the expense then go to the market and the Co-op. As we return, Harry comes puffing up the hill on his rusty old bike, "Got to catch the bank before 12.30pm … (gasp!) … the fuel dock won't accept a card. Goodbye again!"

When *Simetra* leaves its berth to fuel up, of course, it is the attendant's lunch break and siesta. They are still waiting to leave at 3.15pm when we go for our walk, climbing uphill and along a dirt track, to be charged at by a belligerent billy goat. The cliffs are so beautiful, like an extensive rockery ablaze with colour, and wafting the scent of honeysuckle and verbena.

From the headland, we see Harry leaving at 4pm. Poor chap, by the time

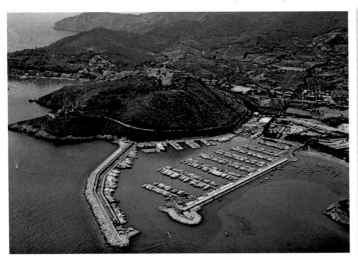

he is two miles off there is a goodly crack of thunder, sending us back in the rain. At 6pm Harry is back in the marina, not caring for the thought of a thunderstorm up his stern all the way down to Capri.

Cala Galera

May 21st Cala Galera to Riva di Triano marina

A local fisherman tells us that summer will not start until after May 20th. Today is fine and clear, so he could be right.

With the usual charming disorganisation, the girl in the office has mislaid our invoice, so we have an unexpected bonus of a free night. We are ready to leave the marina at 9am.

In radio contact with Harry, we hear that he has further delay because of a broken wire on his navigation aid. Further contact with Harry says that he has just been chased and caught by the customs launch, but now at last he is on his way to Greece. He does not seem to be having much luck lately.

On a calm sea, in a light breeze with several dolphins swimming alongside and diving under the bow giving a delightful performance, a little confidence begins to seep back, we relax and enjoy! A few more puffs of wind stir at 1.30pm and we can drift gently along with the jib and mizzen sails. Civita Vechia is in view, and so are its tall red and white striped belching chimneys, fuel tanks and cranes. We can give that a miss!

At 3.20, after 34 miles, we enter an immense new marina and are promptly spotted by the *ormeggiatori*, (attendants), who direct and assist us to berth, then present us with a glossy brochure and poster. The artist's impression looks most inviting, so we cycle off to investigate the showers, shops, bar, supermarket and gardens as illustrated, only to find they have not actually been built yet, so in reality, we are on a building site in the middle of nowhere. There is a tiny shop about a mile down the road, the dockside is too high to get off the boat without a boost from behind, it takes an almighty leap to get back on again, there is a constant slop from the swell and it is more expensive, at £21 per night. Mustn't grumble, anything is better than the wall at St Stephano.

At dusk, the pied wagtails keep us amused as they line up and come to roost under the pontoon at the stern.

May 22nd

Since the only completed showers are half a mile away, I opt for a much nearer Portacabin. It is basic but clean, with plenty of hot water, so I take full advantage to wash a few shirts and towels. By the time a fourth man has come in looking a bit taken aback and embarrassed, it slowly dawns that this is the builder's facility and not for visitors, but I just smile at them until the washing is done.

Meanwhile, Sam has re-organised the taps ready for a hot water system, and washed off the St Stephano mud from the anchor and chain.
There has not been a cloud all day so hopefully the fisherman is right. Should we have sailed today instead of house keeping on an expensive building site?

The wagtails line up again at twilight, waiting to fly one at a time to their roost under the pontoon. There seems to be an order of rank.

The swell persists, slopping the body side to side when trying to sleep.

May 23rd Riva di Triano to Fiumicino

Half past four in the morning, wide awake and twitching about leaving, calling each other 'wimps' as further sleep evades us. The atmospheric pressure has dropped ten millibars during the night - I think I am developing 'Barometer tapper's claw'.

By 8.30am we have washed up, watered up, paid up and are ready to go.

Why is it such a strain to hold the bowlines? It is only because Sam has accidentally left the engine running in slow reverse gear, resulting in me leaping from dock to boat, something that Nureyev would have been proud of.

As expected, there is a tedious slight swell and we are grateful that neither of us is prone to sea sickness. With a light breeze we make good progress across the long featureless bay just ahead of a mass of murky clouds. If the wind increases, it will be difficult to enter the river at Fiumicino, and then it is a further 20 miles to the next port. The 29 miles already is enough for today!

There is a remarkable current sweeping out of the river mouth, a tributary of the Tiber, which has two lifting bridges, one for traffic and the other a footbridge.

The pilot book gives 2.30pm as an opening time so, fighting the flow, a hasty lasso catches a rusty iron barge to hang onto and we wait and wait, for another non-event. The only signs of life are two workmen waiting for the glue to dry on some rubber matting.

Enquiring gestures are mimed, and their shrug is interpreted as, 'Whenever', which happens to be not until 4.30pm, when both bridges go up together. There is plenty of space along the walls, but we have been warned that boats on the town walls are fair game for thieves, so we make our way further along to a small, unimpressive boatyard where help is given to tie up, third boat out from a slimy iron ladder against a high, slimier wall. It feels passably secure, together with a few other cruising boats all sharing the sounds of low flying aircraft as they land and take off from close by Rome airport every two minutes.

May 24th Fiumicino

This is not an attractive place, so it is not the intention to stay longer than necessary to see a bit of Rome. Across the river, a fisherman tends his 'scoop nets', the birds are singing, a wiry little Irishman on the next boat sandpapers his topsides midst a cloud of dust, which settles on the fast-flowing water already coated with white fluff from the trees.

All quite peaceful but we need food and must go to the bank first. What a palaver that is. By the time the automatic doors admit us, we are devoid of all our belongings including watches, belts and penknife, which have to be locked in a cupboard in the foyer. After queuing for fifteen minutes holding up our trousers, the teller, in an open necked shirt over a very off white T-shirt and a cigarette in the corner of his mouth, becomes very flustered in his attempt to deal with our Eurocheque. He flashes a smile when, at last, he masters the transaction. More than expected is spent in the supermarket, and that is the whole morning taken up with bank and shop.

Not having heard of Ostia Antica before, the leaflet makes it sound interesting, but we left it a bit late in the afternoon before deciding to go by bus to look at it. What an experience that is! The bus hurtles at great speed, then stops suddenly every few minutes. The fact that the seats are shiny plastic, lengthways down the sides, there is the imagined prospect of ending up on someone's knee or on the floor.

Changing buses in Ostia town causes an argument between well-meaning other passengers as to which number bus we should take next. As a consequence, we arrive at Ostia Antica too late to embark on the vast extent of the ancient ruins that might take at least three hours to skim through.

After a brief browse round the ancient village and its 15th century Castello, we make the same slip-sliding bus journey back, feeling as if we have been through a mangle. It is certainly worth another visit though.

Can it be that so many Italian bus drivers are thwarted racing drivers?

May 25th

This is a marathon day out with mixed experiences.

Loaded up with camera, umbrella, lunch, water, and a phrase book, we catch the 9.35am train to Ostiense station in Rome, then take the Metro (B line) from Pyramid to Termini, then change to A line for Ottoviano, as instructed.

The Metro is uncomfortably crowded, everyone is crushed up together, and being only five feet and one inch tall, I cannot reach anything to hold onto while the train speeds and stops sharply, the same as the buses, so Sam grabs me now and again. He then makes an awful discovery that his wallet has gone. A man pushes past in a hurry to get out and there is nothing we can do about it, although I did have a chunter, "I TOLD you to put it in the bag!" Most of the time, his hand had been over his wallet deep in his front pocket, but on one extra sharp lurch, when it seemed as if everyone might fall into a heap, he grabbed for the handrail with one hand and for me with the other. In those few moments it had gone! Distressingly, it contains credit cards, driving licence, and £50 worth of Lira.

The crowd explodes onto the platform at Ottoviano with us in the midst, feeling very annoyed with ourselves, upset and trembling, not a good start to what is meant to be a lovely day out.

It is Saturday, therefore no banks are open to cancel the cards and we cannot find a police station to report the loss - they will only laugh, anyway.

We proceed as intended and make our way to the Vatican, where a most imposing staircase in bronze relief leads up to the ticket office. Fortunately, I have my purse and £5 each seems a very fair price for what is to come. There are roughly seven kilometres of rooms and corridors filled with treasures, which include sculptures by Michelangelo and Bernini, huge paintings by Raphael and Botticelli, tapestries on the walls, mosaic floors and ceilings of marble that is patterned, carved, gilded and painted. Your eyes are so overwhelmingly bombarded with colour and spectacle that it is difficult to absorb it all.

The floor of the Sistine Chapel is virtually bare, except for the rapt tourists gazing up in wonder with hushed reverence at the glowing colours of Michelangelo's ceiling. No photography is permitted, you can only stand, or sit on the floor and stare.

In complete contrast, we eat our sandwiches in a very modern snack bar within the building!

When the Vatican closes at 2pm, everyone heads for St Peter's Square - follow the flow! It is not a pretty square, just vast, but with the aid of a guide book we can appreciate the sculptures.

Inside St Paul's Basilica, everything seems of immense proportions. 100ft columns, and the Michelangelo dome that you can go up into, but the queue for the elevator is too daunting. The smaller domes are also splendidly frescoed, but one of the most beautiful sculptures by far, is the famous Michelangelo *Pieta*, it makes you want to reach out and touch it, but sadly it is now behind glass and some distance away.

By late afternoon, the eyes and brain have had a surfeit of wonderment and can take no more for today.

Although weary, another half hearted attempt is made to find a police station by trying to follow directions from two 'Polizia', but with no success. After taking two wrong turns, we find Ostiense station to return to Fiumicino where, instead of just crossing the road back to *Kalivala*, we walk a mile down the road to the local Polizia to report our robbery. That causes a stir!

Directed upstairs, we go to the Superintendent, as he knows two or three words of English. He asks for Sam's passport. Successfully miming, 'Well, we ain't going to walk a mile there and a mile back to fetch it – señor,' Sam is escorted back in a police car driven by an underling who is a bit peeved because he is about to go off duty, whilst I am held hostage until his return.

When all the forms are duly completed in triplicate, and stamped, they happily shake hands all round, then another cheeky little mime portrays, 'How about a lift back again, per favore, señor?' This succeeds and we arrive back in style in the police car. The peeved one is now appeased as he gets a lift home too. There are more smiles, hand shakes and *arriverdercis* – I think they have enjoyed the diversion!

It is now 7.45pm and we are quite limp, but manage to telephone our eldest son to ask him to cancel the credit cards and arrange a new driving licence.

May 26th

Now we must accept that we cannot leave this slimy wall and treacherous ladder until we receive the new credit cards and driving licence, so we take time to look at the other boats and go for a walk.

We meet Frank and Jane from California. Their boat is named after a Scottish island to which they eventually hope to sail and they invite us over for a glass of wine this evening. The rest of the walk is hum-drum: a motorway, another boatyard, and a few large buildings that, at one time had been quite grand but are now derelict.

At 6pm we climb down another ladder to pick our way carefully across the deck between dozens of plastic cans of water, pots of herbs, a vine in a bucket, piles of rope and the anchor chain. Frank and Jane, a charming couple are world cruisers, both over seventy years old and the experiences they recount make us feel bigger cowards than ever. At one particular time, they had been adrift in the Indian Ocean for seven weeks after a storm had left them without steerage or radio. They were battened down for three days. Frank had then rigged the rudder with ropes and they were able to make very slow progress towards land. Meanwhile, their family had presumed them lost at sea after three weeks without news. We are quite humbled.

As we enjoy the wine, they have other visitors from a boat moored further up the river. They are two Americans, a psychologist and his lawyer friend who are busy writing a new pilot book before returning to San Diego, but as they have been away for ten years already, they are not in any hurry.

The conversation is interrupted by a loud splat, much splashing and urgent shouting from a man on top of the wall. The cause of this panic is a large

Alsatian dog which has fallen off the wall and is now desperately swimming round in circles. Concerted efforts eventually drag the poor frightened animal out, and with difficulty, manoeuvre it up the ladder, wetting its rescuers through.

The thankful handler explains that this has happened a few times because the dog is old, has arthritis, is almost blind – and also happens to be the boatyard's watch dog. Some watch dog, you have to watch the dog.

May 27th
Whilst waiting for mail, we resign ourselves to the surroundings and the slimy ladder. An electrical engineer is located for the refrigerator motor, he too just shrugs, and suggests a new one at £500 but we haven't quite given up on it yet!

On a fine, sunny morning we take the train to Rome again but this time my purse is pinned to the inside of my bag, and Sam has a pouch on a string inside his trousers tied to goodness knows where. To avoid the Metro, we walk from the station passing the Baths of Caracalla (built between AD 212 and 217), where The Three Tenors had their concert just last week. It looks most interesting, but 27 acres of it might take a rather long time to visit, so we continue to the Arch of Constantine (AD 315), then on to the Colosseum (AD 80) which is surprisingly without charge unless you want to go upstairs. It is sufficient to just stand and gaze at the sheer size of it, the architecture and the thoughts of all that happened here with the chariot races, gladiators, lions and Christians, and the mock sea battles. The atmosphere is hushed as if one senses the bloodshed and the ghosts of the dead, so it is a relief to come back into the sunshine to walk through paths of roses in Traiano Park to the church of San Pietro in Vincoli where stands the magnificent marble sculpture of Moses by Michelangelo. In a glass case nearby, are reputed to be St Peter's chains. Who knows?

The lady in the church card shop recommends that we see the Basilica of St Maria Maggiore (AD 432 – 440). Here we see ancient Christian mosaics and a spectacular ceiling said to be gilded with the first gold brought from Peru. In a small marble chapel displayed in a gilded case, lies what is believed to be part of Jesus's crib. Again, who knows?

There is such a wealth of frescoes, finery and gold that the mind becomes bedazzled and runs out of superlatives. This is the time to sit on the steps of a fountain, eat our sandwiches midst the pigeons, and reflect on all we have seen.

The walk towards the famous Spanish Steps is interspersed with surprise antiquities, noting that the Palace of Barberini is now an art gallery. On arriving at the Medici Villa, we find that we are at the top of the steps not the bottom as expected. Before descending, we stroll through the pleasant gardens of Villa Borghese, Rome's largest public park with its grand panorama over the domes and spires of the city.

The steps are not as pretty as anticipated, having no flowers on them as shown on all the postcards, and part of them are barricaded off and under repair, but the general atmosphere is pleasing.

At the bottom of the steps is yet another famous sculpture, Baraccia Fountain (Fountain of the Ugly Boat) by Bernini's father in the 17th century, which despite it age, looks quite modern. For a short while we join the horde of other tourists just sitting and people-watching while we rest our feet. How I would love to cool then in the fountain. A nearby McDonald's has been recommended to us for their toilet facilities, but we fail to find it. The Trevi Fountain is also under repair and cordoned off, so we just make our own wish to return to see more of this great city.

The day of the barbecue is warm and sunny. Sam charges up his razor with the generator, while I forage in the market then prepare a salad. At mid-day, assembled on a small patio near the boatyard office are ten assorted cruising crews, including the two Americans, a couple from a village close to our home, Frank and Janet and the organisers.

Through the smoke a very convivial, social three hours pass exchanging experiences until the wine runs out and the embers turn to white ash. Frank is having a problem with his electrics, so Sam and he go off to attempt to solve it. This takes far longer than thought, having to almost re-wire the whole boat in order to stop Janet needing to wear rubber gloves when using her computer. She is writing a cookery book.

May 30th
Today we are invited for tea on the American boys' boat so the bikes are carried over the other two boats and dragged up the ladder onto the dockside. It is a flat ride past an archery and a riding school, then over two miles along a bumpy, pot-holed road beside fields and little houses with meticulous kitchen gardens to find their 44ft *Peterson* yacht moored on the river bank. It is a very well-found craft, although down below it does resemble an office. Tea making is not their strong point, but the conversation flows for an hour over the mugs of anaemic, milky, warm fluid. I'm glad I did not ask for it weak.

On our return, we are invited onto *Isle of Barra* by Janet and Frank at 8pm where, from two seats in the gloom we watch a video film of *Dirty Rotten Scoundrels* featuring Michael Caine. Still mistrustfully wearing her orange rubber gloves, Janet gives us a tub of freshly popped corn to authenticate being at the movies – American style! The pop corn is washed down with some audacious local plonk which compensates for the film not being as funny as expected, but at least it is a pleasant change from reading.

This was to be the first of several evenings spent at the 'movies', the next night being a South African film titled *The Gods Must Be Crazy* which we had never heard of, but it is both charming and very amusing, set in the wilds of Africa. Not so good is its sequel and the nights we quietly suffer *Three Men and a Baby* and *Music Man* along with the popcorn.

A few more days pass with no sign of our mail. We try to find a hotel to telephone from, but I don't think anyone ever wants to stay in Fuimicino so we ask at the boat yard office. That is a mistake and a lesson learnt, as they charge us £12 for a three minute call.

We also learn that if you buy a large flagon of wine at the supermarket, it can be decanted into three of your own bottles out in the car park. The flagon can then be returned to reclaim the money charged on it without delay.

It is still difficult to find nice fresh bread that does not have the shell of a tortoise.

June 1ˢᵗ Fiumicino

Has summer come at last? There has been no rain or thunderstorms for ten days, so taking advantage of the fair weather, we again take the early train into Rome and the Metro to the Coliseum.

The entrance fee to the Forum should be £10, but on trying to translate the notices at the ticket office, learn that it is free for the over sixties. I just point to our grey hair and we are nodded through.

By the time we are less than a quarter of the way round it is obvious that we need a better guide book. We talk to other visitors who have maps, but they are just as confused because many sections are not labelled. The whole vast area is fascinating, particularly the amazing precision of the brickwork.

Lunch is eaten under pine trees in a small garden overlooking the Coliseum, the Triumphal Arch of Titus and the Forum, before descending flights of steps from a Belvedere to a fountain, then down again to temples, arches, basilicas, and the House of the Vestal Virgins. Here I am very tempted to pose on an empty plinth in line with the other statues of ladies, but decorum prevails! There are pieces of carved marble, broken columns and other relics strewn around the ground, and some areas are closed to the public because of the continuing and seemingly endless excavations.

Out of the Forum, an uphill climb comes to Piazza Venezia, then down to pass St Peter's prison. Everywhere you look there are churches, palaces, basilicas and yet more ruins. By mid afternoon we are flagging so sit on a wall watching the world go by when our attention is drawn to four street urchins trying out their pick-pocketing skills on an awestruck posse of black-socked, camera-decked American tourists. Observing this with amusement, we see the targeted man become aware of one of them, turn and give a goodly clout across the ear of a little boy about six years old, who runs off crying back to the other three, who look like older sisters. No sympathy from them, they scold him severely and deal out a further clouting. The way they operate is to wave a magazine or newspaper in front of you to distract you, two then touch or jostle you whilst the fourth one picks your pocket. It is very intimidating, as we well know having experienced the same thing earlier today, fortunately without loss this time!

It is just coincidence that tonight's film on *Isle of Barra* is appropriately *A Funny Thing Happened on the Way to the Forum* – the Michael Crawford version has some good stunts! "Oh, no. Not more popcorn."

June 3rd

An inadequate, not to scale leaflet is studied to try and estimate the distance by road to Ostia Antica, as the eight miles stated does not seem correct. Across the boats and up the ladder again with the bikes. Our plan is to set off and see how long it takes to reach a distance which is marked on the leaflet, which we estimate to be a third of the way, then turn back if it seems too far.

The first stretch is on a motorway, which is a bit unnerving along with all these Italian drivers, but it only takes ten minutes to reach our third of the way point, so within 35 minutes we are at the site entrance.

The fee should have been £4, but the grey hair ploy is accepted and again it is *Gratuito*, for which we thank the Ministry of Culture for so respecting their elders and leave them in charge of the bikes. The next three hours are spent browsing through the Roman streets. This vast area was once the Port of Ostia, a township of 100,000 population during the period between 400BC and around 400AD, until the river silted up and changed its course. Malaria then decimated the people.

The site was not discovered until 1909 and excavations are still in progress. The state of preservation of some of the buildings is remarkable, as is the precision of brickwork and stonework, especially the theatre, although the marble seats might strike a bit cold under the toga.

It is much easier to visualise the layout here than at the Forum in Rome, as the tree-lined streets are all named, boards give information in three languages, and much more of the buildings remain intact. There are colleges, warehouses built round a pillared courtyard lined with shops and surprisingly, blocks of apartments, and a fire station because of the grain stores. Down one street is the *Thermopolium*, which is a bar with a marble counter where hot drinks were served. In places, the original wall paintings are preserved together with the mosaic floors in the houses.

The Forum Baths are the largest of the three bath houses, where the heating ducts, pipes and fire places can still be seen as well as an exercise room and recesses in the walls for togas and sandals, i.e. lockers! Adjacent, much to our amusement and great admiration of these Romans, we locate three very fine 20 holer public latrines, which are almost more civilised than some of the present day French ones. Each room is about four metres square with a channel all round and drainage underneath, two rooms have marble thralls and the other is of stone – perhaps for those of more humble rank! All very clever, and you can just picture them in a row with togas hitched up as they read *The Daily Tiber Tribune*.

It is impossible to do more than just skim through these extensive ruins in one afternoon and as we wander back, we realise that we have not seen any other visitors; it feels a bit eerie as if in a different time zone. Ostia

Antica is well worth another visit one day, a shame the gift shop had no postcards.

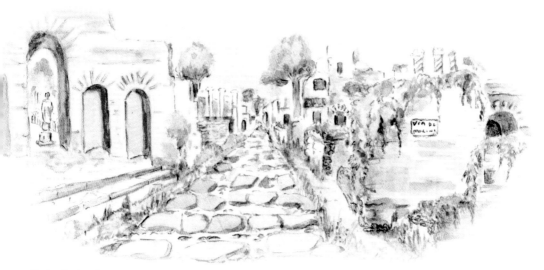

Ostia Antica Street

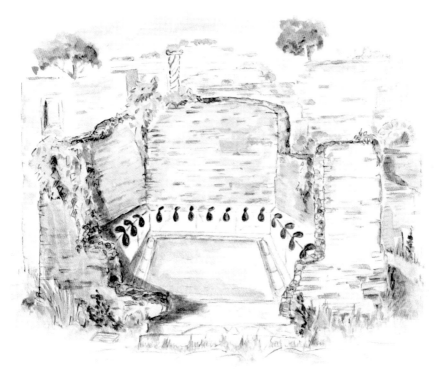

Roman public toilets

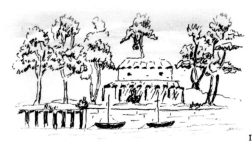

June 4th

A perfect day for sailing, but what has happened to our Express Mail? Several people have recently delighted in relating horror stories about the postal system three weeks, six months, or never!

Having now seen Rome and Ostia Antica, which was the main reason for coming to Fuimicino, we are more than ready to leave this uncharismatic town, in spite of the friendly boat people nearby with their invitations to tea, wine and the nightly film show. How much more popcorn can a body take?

June 5th

On this fair sunny morning, our long awaited letter arrives and we are relieved to find the new credit cards and an insurance claim form, but no driving licence form. The claim form is filled in and posted at once, then we pay the mooring fees so that we can leave next morning at 7.30am when the bridges are raised. The letter also tells us of our eldest son and family's wish to join us for two weeks holiday at the end of June, when they will be flying to Naples. This news evokes mixed reactions of excitement and anxiety about being there in time, as there are still over a hundred and fifty miles to go. Sam begins to worry about Naples and our friendly Italian alongside knows nothing about it either. There is much to do however, stowing bicycles, topping up the water tanks, a dash to the supermarket and saying our goodbyes. Our Italian friend shows us some nice places to go, but they mostly appear to be fine weather anchorages which we now distrust.

We wish we could feel confident about where to meet Paul, Sally, and the two boys, it is spoiling the pleasure of the anticipation.

June 6th

No need for an alarm clock after all. The sound of a south-easterly, force six wind howling up the river woke us at 6am. "No point in ploughing into that," we agree and turn over to sleep until a more sociable hour.

On hearing a shout from the top of the wall, we are surprised to see a friend who we met on Elba. They had arrived yesterday and are moored between the bridges. The gas runs out as we try to make him a cup of tea, and before the cylinder can be replaced we must go to the bank, where there is the usual farce trying to appease the automatic doors to let us in. This time it is the zip on my jacket and the metal clasp of my purse they object to. Luckily they ignored the zip on my jeans. It is a long wait for the same teller as before, who had difficulty in remembering what to do with a Eurocheque, but he does manage to force a smile at last.

There is a good market today, so I leave Sam to be traumatised in Loui's the barber and lose myself amongst the colourful stalls of tomatoes, spices, tomatoes, herbs, tomatoes, a few vegetables and yet more tomatoes.

The wind blows hard all day and the noise from the landings and taking off at the airport every few minutes is deafening and irksome until evening, when Janet is once again popping her corn, while we are falling asleep in front of a very unfunny American CIA spoof film.

June 7th

No plans to leave today either, although the wind has eased slightly, it is now lashing with rain. *Kalivala* is inspected and deemed, mouse free by Bijou, one of the boat cats. A camel walks across the bridge, I wonder why? Is the circus in town?

At mid day, an American yacht comes through the bridge. After helping them moor up and giving them a hot drink to help them recover from a harrowing thrash over from Corsica, we are pondering about five-mile hops.

There is not much else to do in the afternoon except read and listen to the rain and aeroplanes, then make an early start on an Italian recipe found on the back of a packet of pasta, which seemed to lose something in translation.

A lively birthday party diverts us for the evening, well attended by several of the visiting boat crews and a welcome change from the movies. We have a very unsteady splosh back to our respective crafts.

June 8th

Shall we ever be able to get away from this unpretty place? A walk to the end of the wall shows that the sea is definitely uninviting, even the fishing boats are three deep against the wall whilst their owners glumly tend their nets. Just in case there is a chance to sail tomorrow, we buy another flagon of wine to decant in the car park and so claim the 80 pence rebate.

Thunder clouds pass over all day bringing bursts of torrential rain then giving way to a beautiful evening however, the safe moorings and convivial company compensate well for the capricious weather – there is always tomorrow!

June 9th

At 6.30 am the scene is calm and sunny, and I am impatient to get away. Sam is still anxious, even though the barometer has risen from 995mb to 1012; he is not happy.

It is just as well that we did not aim to catch the 7.30am bridge opening. We had forgotten that it is Sunday and the bridge is not opened until 9am.

There is a slight lack of harmony between us during breakfast, so I leave Sam with the washing up to walk down to look at the state of the sea. He is right. It is still very disturbed. I adjust my thoughts towards food for the Sunday barbecue with a much more agreeable attitude.

The ebb current of this stretch of river after the rain takes many diverse objects along its seaward flow. During coffee break we watch with interest the surging by of a huge tree trunk - at least 25ft long and 18 inches in diameter, a burst football, an unreachable fender, cans, bottles, bamboo canes, dead fish, a bloated rabbit and numerous used appliances of which the Pope does not approve.

The barbecue is well attended by sixteen assorted English, American, Canadian and Scottish off-shore cruising groups, all waiting like ourselves, to be on their way again.

By 4pm, the combination of a surfeit of sun, food, wine and endless gossip becomes just tooooo soporific!

June 10th Fiumicino to Nettuno marina

At 5am we are awake, fidgeting, wondering and hoping. The sun in a clear blue sky looks promising as the lines are cast and we circle around waiting for the road bridge to open at 7.30am. As we pass through, the footbridge ahead is just closing, "Oh, bother," or words to that effect, are proved unfounded, as it re-opens a few minutes later to let us out into the sea. It is very choppy but we assume that once clear of the nasty little over-falls near the entrance, it will calm down. Wrong. Wind on the nose with a steep, confused swell so typical of the Mediterranean.

We test it for two uncomfortable miles, then agree that five or six hours more of this tedious motion will not be much fun. Once more cowardice prevails and we return to hang off a rusty barge to wait for the bridge to open again.

There is time for a browse round the market and a few more differences of opinion follow when we see *Isle of Barra* and *Oyster* pass by at mid day. I try to convince myself that their boats are bigger than ours, and we are not really chicken-hearted, just over-careful.

A radio call to *Oyster* assures us that the swell has eased considerably now, so at 12.30pm we are on the way again at last.

The main sail gets an airing but to save time, we have some help from the engine, and at 6pm, after 27 miles, we arrive alongside of *Oyster* at Nettuno, another new, expensive and unappealing marina.

June 11th Nettuno to San Felice Circio

After waiting twenty minutes at the fuel dock, the man in the tower shouts to say that it is closed, so we leave, setting a course for Capo Circio, which is just discernible in the distant mist. When less than a mile off-shore, a large power boat comes tearing towards us, making no attempt to alter course, then suddenly stops alongside. Pirates perhaps? No, police. What have we done wrong? We did pay the marina fees.

Very officiously we are instructed to alter course to 216 degrees for six miles because of naval and military exercises in operation in this area. This takes us considerably off-course and Cap Circio disappears completely, so we cheat a little and steer 200 degrees for five miles instead, waiting for the action to begin. A few dull thuds are duly heard, then five motor torpedo boats race each other down the bay and that is it. It seems an endless time before the Cap becomes clear again. This headland is said to have once been the home of the enchantress Circe, with whom Ulysses dallied for a year.

After having to motor sail for most of the 29 miles, the wind arrives from nowhere just in time to make an embarrassment of mooring up in the marina where we have to resort to going in bow-to.

The surroundings are pleasant, with the historic village up a steep hill. Walking back down with bottles of really cold beer and six eggs, the strap on my bag suddenly snaps. Why does it have to be the bottles that smash, not the eggs?

June12th San Felice Circio to St Antonio

In the doorway of the nearest little shop, the careworn matriarch sits on an orange box, arms folded as she waits for custom, then expectantly follows us inside and hovers hopefully. 'Sorry to disappoint you señora, but row upon row of tinned tomatoes and packets of every shape pasta is not what I want.'

It is well worth the steep climb back up into the delightful old village to sit with a coffee in the square and to be dazzled with the riot of hot colours of the bougainvillea, next to the brilliant nasturtiums and hydrangea that bedeck the walls.

There is quite a lot to see around here, if you have a car, said the girl with flashing dark eyes at the Information Office. There are caves, ruins, a lighthouse and a nature park, which has a hot area on one side of the mountain and a cold area on the other, but not within our reach I regret.

On our descent, we have a sudden urge to move on whilst the weather is favourable, and it is an uneventful twenty-three mile sail, in spite of Sam looking suspiciously over his shoulder at the one black cloud in the distance and imagining an increased swell. The usual blast of wind greets our arrival at St Antonio, near Gaeta.

The first harbour is as exposed as St Stephano, so we quickly exit and continue to the Yacht Club marina, where seeing no-one to direct us, we nose into the first empty berth we see. That soon brings a man running down the pontoon, who tells us that for the privilege of this place with no water or electricity (and tepid showers) we have to pay £28, but it is too late now.

In compensation, it is a pleasant town. There are good shops close by with a proper butcher where we buy excellent pork chops, but at this price, we must move on again tomorrow.

June 13th St Antonio to Formia
Leaving at 9.30am we hope to find a space in nearby Gaeta harbour. It is full and very exposed, so we motor along the coast for another three miles to Caposele, which looks a good area. Only minutes after mooring up, we are politely thrown out by a gold-braided buff declaring that the harbour is full.

The next place along the coast is Formia, a commercial and fishing port, which has a large expanse of harbour that also seems to be full. Hoping to see an *Ormiggatore* to help, we motor round, hear a shout and see a man beckoning. He is moving his dinghy to make a space for us and then kindly takes our lines. This is not a very salubrious haven, but it is free and we are grateful to have a safe mooring.

As advised, we report to the *Capitano's* office which causes the usual flutter when another young sailor gets some practice writing in the 'big book', as they are not very used to having visiting foreign yachts - this is fisherman's territory.

The evening scene is lively with the constant passing of the locals - some on their way to fish from the wall carrying gallon canisters of wine, a stool, and all their tackle, while the mothers and children slowly primp by in their finery, stopping to say *Ciao*. They seem curious about this lone English yacht midst all the fishing boats.

Later, all the boats go out to fish for pilchards and sardines with the bright lights on the bows, the men all shouting to each other as they go. Some return at 1am, others at 5am still shouting - quite a busy night for all.

June 14th
It is hot, humid and our corner reeks of dead fish that are thrown overboard when the fishermen clean their nets - still shouting and joking with each other. They are very friendly to us with offers of fish, which regretfully, are tactfully refused since I do not care for gutting, or the smell in the cabin.

The Tourist Office plies us with books, but most places of interest are further away than a comfortable bike ride, and all uphill. At noon we hear numerous explosions and assume it is from another naval exercise, then we see a succession of fireworks at the end of the pier, each one the same and almost invisible against the bright sunlight, but giving off palls of thick smoke. No-one seems to know the reason unless it is for the bride and groom seen earlier at the restaurant, who are now lost in the smoke.

Another *grosso* flagon of cheapo plonk is bought, then this time we decant it in the supermarket doorway and get back £1.40. Wow. Then Sam breaks a tooth on some 'doorstep' bread at lunchtime. He receives a very prompt appointment from a nearby dentist, which costs £150. "Well, it is porcelain, señor." And we thought that the money back on the flagon was a bonus.

Looking round the town there is *Torre di Molo*, a Roman fortification with a moat and a 1200 tower, both under renovation. In the same street, many buildings have shell holes and damage sustained in World War ll, when much of the town was demolished by American and British troops. Most has since been, not too sympathetically rebuilt.

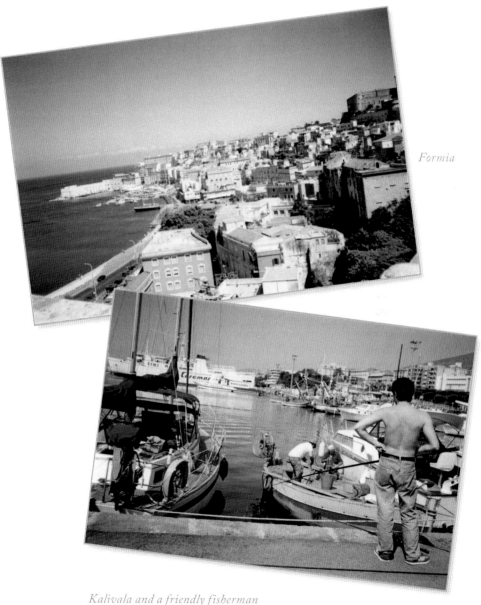

Formia

Kalivala and a friendly fisherman

*June 15*th

Hot, humid and smelly again, but we are becoming immune to the stench of the festering fish. Produce in the market is now better quality and cheaper, although still expensive by English prices.

Walking uphill, we come to an ancient tower and the church of St Arasmo. Both are closed so we wander back down and along the beach at Vendicio, passing by the remains of Cicero's Villa, also closed and neglected. There are so many interesting, ancient sites just crumbling away and ignored, but then this is not a tourist area.

The steamy heat is tiring, we sit under the cool umbrella pines to eat our picnic lunch - the beers are now warm, the bees drone and we shall fall asleep if we don't move down to the beach. Sitting on the gravel beach is not comfortable, but we stay long enough to have the first swim of the summer. The sea is surprisingly warm, not crystal clear but sufficiently refreshing to face the three-mile walk back.

Evening entertainment is from the passing fashion parade and dolled-up children watching us watching them until 9.30pm, when the fishermen start shouting as they set out. Later, security lights come on overhead and it feels as if we are trying to sleep in the middle of a football stadium - during a match!

*June 16*th

My only thoughts today are about moving on, as we are both becoming anxious to find somewhere more suitable for the family to come for their holiday. This place is so busy at night that you cannot sleep well and also, the two grandsons will need a nice beach to play on.

The hot humidity continues and the locals are rumouring *Sirocco*, so we are not over joyful.

*June 19*th *Formia to Casamicciola, Isle of Ischia*

Despite the disturbed sleep, we are ready to cast off at 8.30am. The fishermen say it is OK, but *poco mosso* - a bit rough. The *Capitano* still says, "Better tomorrow."

Sailing at 6.5 knots we soon reach the residual swell, which is expected.

Now what have we done wrong? The Guardia Finanza (Customs) is pounding after us. With an authoritative flourish, the powerful launch swooshes up alongside, and three gold-braided white suits eye us up and down for a few minutes. After a few words between themselves they salute, wave, hoot and then swoosh, off again leaving a five feet wash to slop across our deck. Perhaps it was a case of mistaken identity.

The slewing motion is tedious, but as it is only 23 miles to this new marina we read about at Pinetemare, we should be there by lunchtime.

How wrong can we be? The now decreasing wind shifts to a head-wind, slowing down progress, so the engine is started to be able to hold course without needing to tack. The waves are higher – not to worry – at last, we can see our intended destination in the distance through the binoculars. On the approach another look shows three blocks of flats, waves breaking over a ruined wall, no masts and no sign of life at all. Later we learn that this so-called, fine new marina had run out of money before it could be finished. Disappointedly, we turn away. Now where?

The swell has increased to two and a half metres on the starboard quarter as we alter course towards the Island of Ischia for another three hours of nauseous rolling. Spirits are low, but soon we are having to concentrate on avoiding ferries in the narrow entrance to the busy Port of Ischia. Circling round and round, seeing just nowhere to moor we are very disheartened and I am ready to cry as we dodge another two ferries on the way out of this crowded harbour.

The pilot book shows another new marina two miles further on. Will it be like the other one and be derelict?

It is a welcome surprise to find that this new marina really does exist, has lots of space and laid lines to pick up for mooring. The resident gust of wind comes promptly to blow us across two anchor chains; *Kalivala* does not answer well to reverse manoeuvres so again, has to go bow to, which is not as easy for access, especially with bicycles.

The *Capitano* is welcoming, but insists that we leave before the weekend as the marina is then full, which we interpret as meaning that it is more lucrative for him to have room for the big power boats from Naples rather than a 32ft yacht for a mere £17.50 per night.

The little town is handy with good shops where we find the nearest thing to bacon yet and, it has a little beach overlooking an odd-shaped rock – Fungi rock. Our spirits recover slightly, but why is there some kind of hassle wherever we go? Sailing is supposed to relieve you of stress. Up to now, we have only made 655 miles of progress, including the 41 today.

June 20ᵗʰ

Since there has not been a water point for over a week, full advantage is taken scrubbing the decks and filling up the tanks without having to lug the five-gallon containers across the dock. Everything here is to hand, but dearer than the mainland. Bus tickets have to be bought from the supermarket and having been told about *Posiedon Gardens*, we take another mad ride to where the bus drops us off at the top of a hill, still two miles away from the gardens that can be seen below looking like a holiday complex.

Agreeing that it does not seem worth the long walk down, we board the next bus that comes along, which stops at the top of another steep hill leading down to Porto Angelo and its small, shallow and crowded harbour.

This is an attractive little town, having several *Termes* hot spring spas with hotel accommodation. From a seat in the square, we watch tourists arrive by the ferry load who head straight for the bar and stay there until the next ferry comes.

It is a long, hot slog back uphill to catch the bus for the return journey. Ischia is not such a pretty island as Elba, being more volcanic and a bit stark.

June 21st Casamicciola to Baia

Tonight, the weekenders will be here in their super luxurious power boats so we have to leave. *Capitano* keeps us waiting while he adds on a few more hundred lire than expected, he has made sure you do not go without paying by keeping the ship's papers until he has thumped the last rubber stamp onto the invoice.

Setting out at 10.40am, we are hoping to stop at the next island, Procida, about seven miles off; an enjoyable passage in spite of a messy sea. As usual, the main port is full unless you wish to hang nose-to-tail on the end of three other boats, just swinging about. That we do not relish, so head back a few miles to the mainland.

Misena does not feel right, most of the boats are small, although there is an anchorage, so we continue round the headland to Baia, where the gestures on the shore are interpreted as, 'Clear off,' so we do. The next bay looks no more promising as we circle round in dismay, not wanting to go any further. There are a few buoys, their slimy green ropes holding a sadly neglected variety of small craft. In the centre of these is the grisly sight of several, half sunken hulls of larger ships, trawlers, or coasters with their rusty broken rigging protruding at all angles. The little bay is exposed and floppy, not a house or sign of life to be seen, it is most eerie but, over there is a vacant buoy!

Picking this up, we hope that its owner will not return tonight and trust that the buoy is heavy enough to hold *Kalivala* from drifting onto this wreckage. Why is it there? Is it more war damage or the result of earthquakes that this area is prone to? Whatever the cause, it is really disquieting and feels like sleeping in a cemetery.

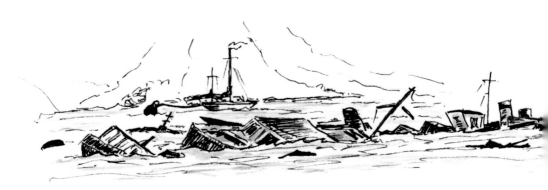

Derelict ships at Baia

June 22nd Baia to Mergellina marina at Naples

The owner did not return, the buoy held firm, the swell subsided and we had a comfortable night, yet there is nothing to keep us here. Letting go of the buoy and cautiously picking our way out, hoping not to become impaled on any under-water wreckage, we take a last look at this strange scene of destruction.

Pozzuola is the next port down the coast and noted for being the birth place of film star Sophia Loren. From a distance, the old Roman town looks agreeable and appears to have masts in the harbour, so the pilot book is checked to look up its amenities. It says, 'The town is at the centre of the volcanic area known as the *Phlegrean Fields* and has suffered on several occasions, from changes in the level of the land, which has affected this region. The harbour, because of its uncertain depths, has been evacuated and is now inhabited by large bold rats.' Well, I think we can give that a miss too – but it might explain the sunken ships in Baia.

Nisida comes into sight on a promontory, almost an island and that seems too small and shallow. On rounding Punta Gaiola, where there are rocks and a navigation beacon, the depth finder suddenly shows only 2.2 metres of water and begins to sound its alarm – and so do we. Head down, hanging over the side, "I can't see the bottom," so the turbulence from a passing ferry is blamed, and Sam does a few reverse thrusts with the motor, which sets it right but trips the log.

After about 12 miles, Naples and its vast marina are seen – it looks quite unappealing. Milling around inside we cannot see a reception quay, just rows of very large power boats, so pull into a vacant space where we are promptly aware of the usual, 'Go away' gestures. We comply and circle, looking for some signs of help but see no one, so now try being cheeky and return to the 'Go away' man for a little argument. This gets results as within minutes, a smart young man comes aboard to take us to an empty mooring then secures the lines and salutes – all very courteous, but there is the feeling that a tip is expected – or is he just being kind?

June 23rd

This city wakes up early, even on Sunday. There are crowds of people, chaotic hooting traffic and Antonio on the next boat is slaughtering *O Solo Mio* - well out of tune, with his too loud radio.

Nearby is a funicular which takes us up to what we thought would be a panoramic viewpoint, but it is just a higher part of town. The long walk down has some interesting glimpses onto the ingenious roof-top gardens and half way down is a square with a more scenic outlook. Here there are wedding groups being photographed but a closer look reveals that who we thought were the brides, are little girls so presumably it is a Confirmation ceremony. Further along, policemen are holding back the strollers to make way for jostling cameramen trying to get the best shots of a glamorous girl in a flamboyant long dress and the Italian equivalent of 'Jack the lad' in an eye-watering red shirt, as they tear to and fro on a scooter.

The parading lasts longer tonight, the little girls have silver balloons and the gathering of macho exhibitionists all have persistent hooters on their scooters, until at some late hour we hear fireworks. The locals have had an exciting day, or is this a normal Sunday?

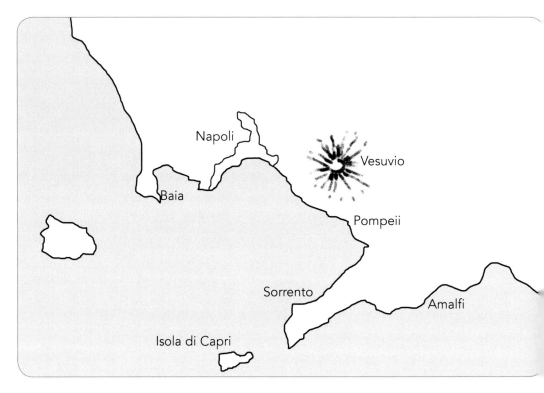

June 24ᵗʰ

It takes longer than usual to find provisions, this is not an area for supermarkets, and we traipse from one tiny shop to another, each one with just a doorway with the daunting matriarch sitting on guard outside. We never did find any Indian tonic.

From high up yesterday we had noticed a beach, but when we find it we learn that it is £2 for an umbrella, £1.50 for a deck chair and £2 just to set foot on it! The umbrella and chair are not priorities, but my Yorkshire roots object to paying to sit on a public beach in spite of the tempting waves, and so we make do with sitting on the rocks on the harbour wall to be splashed.

The children here catch little fishes by making a two-inch hole in the top of a plastic-covered, wide-necked jar, put a bit of flour in the bottom then rub the top with more flour and set it down in just under two feet of water. Then they wait. They were catching several fish every few minutes; it might be worth remembering in case there are gaps in amusing the two boys next week.

June 25th

A nearby railway station has an impressive flight of marble steps and floors from where we take a short ride to the main Garibaldi station and locate the Piazza where the buses leave for the airport, in readiness for the weekend. We are given garbled instructions from a very patient driver who insists on shaking hands as we thank him.

At 10.20am we board the Trans-Vesuvian railway to Sorrento in order to find out the possibilities of a mooring in the marina. It takes one and a half hours to pass through the unexciting landscape of ugly apartments and a few market gardens. By the time the tourist office is located it is closed, as we were diverted by the first sighting of a supermarket.

It is a very steep descent down to the little harbour, where we are inspected by two well-starched, white-uniformed officials only to be told that they have no room for our draught of 1.5 metres.

Sitting next to an English family, we enjoy lunch under the trees before making the long, hot climb back up into the town to wander the streets. Perhaps we did not see it from the best angles, but there is no real desire to *ritorno a Sorrento* again.

Returning, we note that both Pompeii and Herculaneum are on this same railway line, and are nearer to Naples.

June 26th

Not being too happy in this marina, we walk to try and find the other marinas listed, taking care not to tread on the freshly caught octopus that have escaped from their containers onto the pavement.

Musing on Pavarotti singing about *Santa Lucia*, we have great hopes of its marina, which has ideal moorings, attractive surroundings with gardens and a bar. Disillusioned again. Reception is oozing with apathy, saying, "No room," without us even bothering to check – and we have smartened ourselves up too. Further on is the yacht club, which has its own swimming pool but even flashing our very respected club card makes no impression and there is the same reply, albeit with apologies. Next to the yacht club is the *Lega Italie Navale* club where they are most helpful and courteous, but again no luck. Somewhat dejected we realise that we must stay in Mergellina.

It is now very hot in the city so we catch a bus back; a frightful experience. Overcrowded, everyone is packed together when I sense something. I look down to see, at waist height a slim hand with wiggling fingers crossing in front of me towards a man's pocket. How I wish I'd had the presence of mind to grab the slim hand and hold on to it, or jab it with a pin but no, I am transfixed, perhaps only for a few seconds before I give his victim a good push out of the pick pocket's reach, whereupon I get a mistrustful glare. With a sigh of relief we get off the bus two stops before intended.

The hot day has kept the water warm in the hose pipes, making no need to walk the distance to the shower block. Whilst relaxing in the cockpit, we are disturbed by a chrome and Tupperware monster mooring up beside us, blocking out the daylight

June 27th
The next three days are mainly spent cleaning, shopping and trying to make extra space. Asking at the fish dock for ice to boost the lazy refrigerator, I am sent to a van and as I wait, watch how to clean and gut the baby octopus ready for cooking - that stops them from wandering off. A six inch cube of ice is all the ice man can spare, which lasts about half an hour before being reduced to a litre of cloudy water; not a very good idea after all.

No one seems to be able to tell us how far it is to the airport. The time it takes to get there is estimated between five minutes and three quarters of an hour, depending on the traffic, and the distance is answered with a shrug.

In the evenings we join in with the parade on the quay, remarking on the fashions, the size and opulence of the power boats compared to the disgraceful amount of rubbish lying around on the rocky harbour wall. The rocks are patrolled by a gang of scrawny, evil-eyed, mangy, feral cats mostly 'in kit', who search for the countless rats attracted by these piles of bottles, tins and discarded pizzas. The harbour authorities do nothing and appear not to notice although the local people seem to feel shame about their country and its present affairs (1991). Perhaps by now, time will have made many changes.

On the 29th June we wish each other a happy 41st Wedding Anniversary - no cards, no flowers, just a promise to celebrate at some other time as we are both excited and apprehensive about the next two weeks, especially now as the wind pipes up with a spectacular display of lightning over the sea. No doubt we shall have fun, regardless.

June 30th
In the continuing strong wind, we are asked to move to another berth – quite tricky in such a confined space when the wind has more control than our reverse gear, but it is a much quieter position.

A phone call from the family says that their plane will now be landing at 6.30pm instead of 2.30pm. Without thinking to ring the airport to check, we leave at 3pm for the two buses, still not knowing how long it will take. Anticipation turns to disappointment when, on arrival we learn that there is a further two and a half hour delay. Not caring to wait there for another five hours, reluctantly we take the two crowded buses back again, when during the journey, a kindly lady mimes a reminder to keep a close hold onto my handbag. 'Don't worry, dear. I will.'

Never mind the expense, at night always take a taxi we are advised, so Sam arrives back with the exhausted four travellers at eleven o'clock and no one cares how narrow the bunks are.

July 1st

After some early morning chaos when our son Paul, his wife Sally, Tom aged nine and Russell seven, are all trying to get dressed and stow their bedding in the small saloon that is also their bedroom, we are assembled and ready for the 10am train to nearby Herculaneum.

The origins of this ancient city remain vague, but it is thought to have been founded in the 4th century BC and was struck by a torrent of mud flooding down from the slopes of Vesuvius during its eruption in 79AD. Unlike Pompeii, which was engulfed by lava and ash it is much better preserved, giving it a more real atmosphere. Surprisingly, almost all of the inhabitants managed to escape.

Still virtually intact are a bakery, wine shops, the Forum, baths, mosaic-floored villas with brightly coloured paintings of sea food and vegetables, and the *Bordello* with three amazing erotic wall-paintings. The whole site is compact enough to get round in spite of the heat, and our picnic lunch is eaten in the shade, sitting on a house wall in Cardio IV Street. Although the boys show a certain flicker of interest, they are certainly more impressed with the ice creams that follow.

All agree that it has been a tiring but interesting first day. "Come down off those rocks, Russ. It's bedtime."

July 2nd Mergellina to the Isle of Capri

This looks a settled sunny day, let's hope it continues. First, the essentials are dealt with, i.e. a double ration of cash, a flagon of wine and extra food, then we are ready to at last get away from this place. For the first time all weather conditions are just right, and the spiders are blown out of all three sails for a pleasant 16 mile sail.

"Please don't swing on the boom, Russ!" Tom is a little more interested in navigation and the techniques of sailing, and he manages to steer a reasonable course for a short span. "I shouldn't lean quite so far over the bow, if I were you, Russ!"

In time for a late lunch, we arrive at the Marina Grande on Capri to be shown and aided into a berth, welcomed in fact, by white-uniformed officials. What a change from, "No room." Everywhere looks attractive with an air of expense, then we realise the reason for the big welcome. At £45 per night they don't have many customers. We pay for two nights, although the minimum stay is supposed to be three.

Nearby is a small beach where we all enjoy wallowing in 70 degree clear water, before looking around some of the town and noting that the tourist gift shops are not too trashy and prices are surprisingly reasonable.

A taxi driver offers his, *Good price £40, señor* for a trip round the island, which compared to the moorings is cheap! *Domani forse* we tell him.

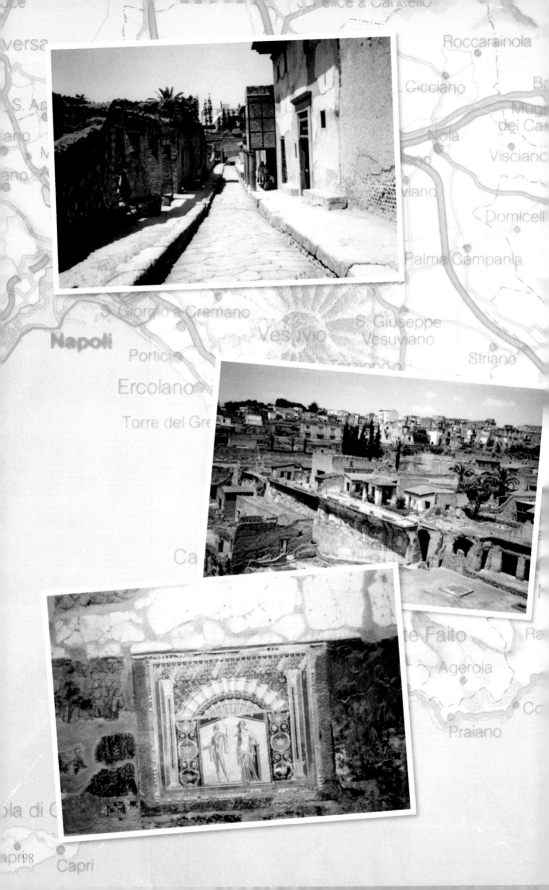

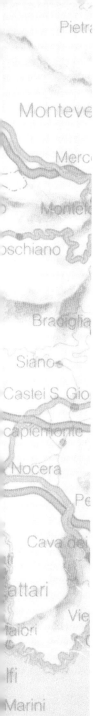

The sun is still glinting through our sun downers as we realise that everything has been on our side today, it has been perfect. "Your cup does not look very safe there, Russ." "Oh dear, never mind."

July 3rd

Blue Italian skies above tra la la...! Although we were warned that it is busy here in the mornings, it is a shock to see so many ferries spilling out swarms of sightseers all heading in the same direction as us towards the funicular up into town, and there is a long queue.

It is a spectacular ascent to the charming square that has restaurants, a clock tower and church. Leading off from here are many small exclusive shops with quite tasteful, fair priced goods on sale – much nicer than expected. Most of the bars and cafés are thronging, so we buy bread, cheeses, tomatoes, fruit and drinks to take to a little park to eat. Having just found a vacant seat for six, we see a notice saying, 'No picnics', which causes a few junior moans. "But I'm hungry NOW!" It is only a short grizzle away to the next park, which has a wonderful view over the bay to be absorbed with lunch, which sustains the boys only as far the square, where ice creams are compulsory.

Back down the funicular, there is time for a swim, a cup of tea and a snack for the ever-hungry boys, before booking the taxi for 4.30pm.

The taxi is a 1950's, open top Fiat 1500, with a blue and white striped awning, six comfortable seats and deemed fab by the lads. The tour of the island is delightful, the driver stops to allow half an hour in Anacapri town before taking us to the base of Monte Solare (589 metres). Here, our individual seats on the chair lift swing us quietly over gardens, terraces and moorland, with our feet almost touching the bushes at times. Twenty minutes of tranquil gliding with only the sounds of the birds, takes us to the top of this small mountain, to be rewarded with an unforgettable panorama over the island and across the sea to the Isle of Ponza.

The descent is equally splendid and even the boys rated it, 'Ace!' They have earned their ice creams for sitting still in the chair lift.

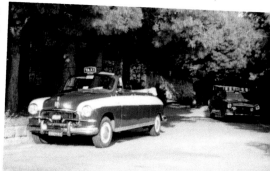

1950's open top Fiat 1500cc taxi

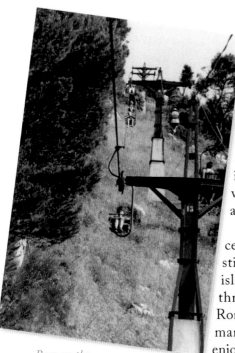

Boys on the Funicular

The driver continues round winding roads to see Gracie Field's house and across to Villa Jovis, which are the ruins of the residence of Emperor Tiberius from 27 to 37AD. Excavations have uncovered servants' and imperial quarters, together with cisterns to supply the baths. Close by is Tiberius's Leap, a precipitous cliff over which he is said to have thrown his enemies, and perhaps some of his wives.

It has been another great day out, we certainly had our money's worth, yet there is still so much more of interest to see on the island, which over the centuries has passed through the domination of the Spanish, Romans, French and English, and has seen many battles. We have only had a brief, but enjoyable glimpse.

July 4th Capri to Isle of Ischia

The Marina Grande is left behind at 9.30am to sail by another famous attraction, The Blue Grotto. Already little boats are queuing up to take the tourists inside on this calm, humid morning. The coastline is sheer and very beautiful, but there is only one anchorage on Capri, as everywhere else is too deep. The Island of Ischia

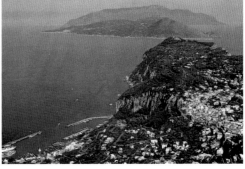

View over Capri town and Marina Grande

is in sight by 11am with Tom on the helm and Russ finding every possible precarious boat part from which to swing. Luckily, we find a buoy to pick up in the lee of a small islet, joined by a causeway to St Angelo. This is ideal for a lunch time break, but now we need to be able to walk ashore to keep everyone amused. Motoring the last few miles of the 21, we enter *Porto D'Ischia* and question our luck at finding a tight space between a smelly fishing boat and an even smellier drain. 'Don't knock it. We have not been thrown out yet, and its free.'

There is a hasty departure for the beach, with ice creams on the way. Without warning, a motorbike, which has been left ticking over, chooses to fall over as I pass by gouging a two-inch area out of my leg. "I didn't touch it, honest." The lady in the ice cream shop is very kind when I return to bleed on her doorstep and she gives me some ice and tissues which help to numb the gouge and stem the bleeding. Having to watch the others swimming is most frustrating.

Paul and Sally join the evening paraders whilst we babysit, wondering whether to breath in the effluence on one side or the fish fumes on the other as we watch the frequent ferries coming and going.

July 5ᵗʰ Porto Ischia to Casamicciola

Having forgotten just how much food children can graze through during a day, another forage is needed before we can leave. It is barely two miles round the headland for our second visit to this place, so we are moored up in good time for lunch, then the family row round to the little beach. We choose to walk, although it is a six man dinghy.

Some grand sandcastle building causes much interest amongst the Italian children, who only seem to play ball in the sea whilst their parents play serious card games under an umbrella. They do not realise that children have to dig and build on English beaches in order to keep warm. Soon, the local children take an interest and begin copying with subsequent rivalry, and great entertainment for the adults until the next feeding time.

Ischa harbour

Kalivala anchored in Casamicciola

Apart from shampooing the boys' hair under the hosepipe and, "Please boys, don't jump over the flower pots, you might knock the heads off the ... Oh dear, you'll have to hide it," we are almost inconspicuous amid the 100ft. sumptuous craft with their uniformed crews.

Yet another ice cream in the sociable little square seems a good way to round off another successful day. Even the strangled rendering of *Santa Lucia* from Luigi the wailing waiter at the opposite restaurant, keeps no one awake.

July 6ᵗʰ Casamicciola to Lacco Ameno

Since there is no chance of staying here for the weekend, we make a quick dash for more food whilst there are good shops. The *Capitano* recommends an anchorage at Cala Mesigna, about three miles away, so at 10.15 am all are ready for off.

It appears that a few dozen other boats also know about it too, mainly motor boats, which make the water very *woppy*, but still nice enough when you can find a space to drop the anchor. Paul takes the boys in the dinghy to explore the rocks and caves, leaving the rest of us to swim, snorkel, sunbathe and sleep. I could get to like this.

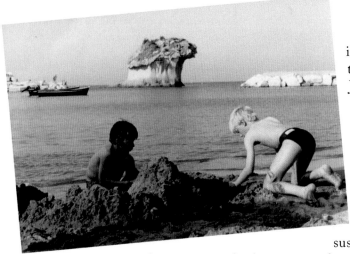

Mid-afternoon and it is time to find somewhere to settle for the evening. Just another few miles on is *Lacco Ameno*, or 'Lack of Amenities' as it becomes named. The first harbour we try gets the usual, "Go away. Privato," but we are told to go to the next one. It's free. To our great surprise, and a little suspicion, here is a very new, almost empty harbour apart from a few fishing boats. The entrance is very shallow and exposed to the north-east, otherwise it is ideal, but we've been caught before, so fingers crossed. The little town is agreeable, with limited shops and has a small beach to play on. After another full day we are quite happy to babysit.

Next day being Sunday, the boats are streaming like lemmings round to the Cala Mesigna, which creates more wallowing than before, prompting the boys to row themselves through an arched rock onto a small gravelly beach and the rest of us swim to it.

Youngsters have a short attention span, so it is back to the lively little square watching the locals enjoy their day off as we wade through yet more ice cream. Running out of ideas for supper we cheat, and collect Pizzas, which are rather more superior than our well-known English ones, thinking they would really quieten the boys' appetites for tonight. Wrong. A later walk seems to require even more ice cream from a different shop; the boys are becoming connoisseurs.

It is slightly disconcerting to notice a vacuous-looking young man just sitting on the dockside gazing down at us until it is almost dark. He watches our every movement, even from the aft hatch you can see this slack expressionless face staring at us. "No problem," say the fishermen. "E's 'armless." We assume that is what becomes of you if you drink too much of this cheap wine.

Fungus rock Casamilliola Ischia

July 8th

There is a beer and soft drink shortage to attend to before going back to the anchorage, which is much quieter today, so we are able to anchor closer to in the bay

A fender is strung from the aft rail for hanging on to, and the boys' swimming and jumping in the sea greatly improves, but Sam regrets fixing up the boarding plank on the side. It was good fun playing at walking the plank until Sally is the unlucky one, and a nasty creaking sound precedes total collapse. That is the end of that game.

An attempt at a siesta fails, as does all our ploys to try and tire the lads out. Where do they get their energy? "You have been told not to jump over the flower pots because you might … Well, we told you so."

Back to *Casamicciola* where there is water and electricity.

July 10th

The weather has settled to hot, hot, hot. Today we catch the bumpy bus into Forio and are surprised to see that there is now a new but unfinished marina, priced at £15 per night, which is quite realistic for this area. The cathedral and town are unremarkable, the Art Exhibition does not lure us past the door, and Paul's attempt to buy swimming trunks causes annoyance. The over-eager salesman becomes very petulant when Paul asks for a smaller size as he does not have any in stock. The salesman turns so belligerent that Paul almost has to fend him off. Trade must be bad. That episode calls for ice creams and drinks at the corner bar where we conclude that, apart from a pretty fisherman's church overlooking steep cliffs and rocks, there is nothing to captivate the attention of two lively lads.

The next bus along is going to St Angelo. We have been before so know there is a beach for the boys at the bottom of the hill, and when they hear that there are ice creams too, the long walk is no problem. It is the drag back up that is exhausting. We still have to play the card game, *Chase the Lady* before bedtime, with the 'funny fellow' looking down the hatch watching every move.

July 11th Lacco Amino to Chialella

There is just enough breeze to waft across to the small island of Procida. First we call in at its marina to book a berth for tonight, then return to a cosy little anchorage off the tiny islet of Vivara we had noticed on the way.

In 15 feet of crystal clear water at 74° F, we splash away the afternoon, loosing all hope of a siesta. It is a nice surprise on our return that the marina had remembered our reservation, but a bit quick to ask for the £20.

The town has just one street of tiny shops, an odd little place but it does have an ice cream shop. Sitting in a small park, while Russ plays on the swings, he has his purse stolen by some children, "Well, you took it off your belt. You can't do that here." It is a hard lesson for a seven-year-old we think as we pacify his sobs.

Back on board, by way of diversion turns are taken to hose down the deck, each of the boys trying to soak the other when, amid the hilarity we find that there is now a swimming pool in the cockpit. The drains are blocked. Up comes the duck-board for much to-do, poking and flushing, which eventually reveals a beer bottle top and some soggy crisps. Although only eight miles have been sailed, it has seemed a very long day.

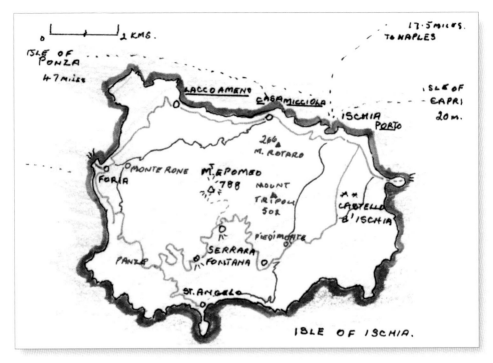

Map labels:
0 ____ 2 KMS.

17.5 MILES TO NAPLES

ISLE OF PONZA 47 MILES

LACCO AMENO

CASAMICCIOLA

ISLE OF CAPRI 20 m.

ISCHIA PORTO

266 M. ROTARO

MONTE RONE

FORIA

M. EPOMEO 788

MOUNT TRIPODI 502

CASTELLO D'ISCHIA

PANZA

PIEDIMONTE

SERRARA FONTANA

ST. ANGELO

ISLE OF ISCHIA.

July 12th Chaialella to Misena

The settled weather thankfully allows us to sail each day, after fetching yet more food. Another pleasant anchorage off Procida town takes care of the afternoon water sports and then we have to start looking for a place for the night.

In Cala Corricella, a very small harbour, we motor round and round looking for the two fishing boats which we had been told allowed you to hang off them. Apparently they were the only possible places but they are nowhere to be seen, so we sail into Procida port. We seem to be in luck here as there is just one space, and two boys, perhaps aged about eleven and thirteen are beckoning us into it. One boy stands on the bow of the boat next to the slot; he is holding a rope, which we presume will be handed to us but as we reverse in, he pulls up the rope until it is fouled under our propeller and rudder. Is this done purposely or in ignorance? We signal for him to lower it, but he just pulls it tighter. There follows a fair measure of shouting and gesturing with no one really sure what the other is saying. Finally, we nudge into place where the boys secure our lines.

Our first thoughts are 'Are they expecting a tip? Because they are not getting one.' The younger lad then, very aggressively demands !0,000 lire. We think that is what he said so we tell him that we are not paying him and want to see the *Capitano*. He then grows very stroppy, No, no. You pay me," then with his fingers, signals 30,000 lire (£15). This does not feel official and more angry words are exchanged and his next gesture is interpreted as '30,000 lire, or we cut your lines.' Is this the junior Maffia at work? We do not stay to find out. It has been a most unpleasant and worrisome encounter.

By now, there is nowhere else we know of to comfortably stay on Procida, so most reluctantly make a choppy passage back to the mainland, to an anchorage at Nisena that has previously been disregarded. It is twelve miles away, well sheltered and reassuring to see another English yacht already anchored there. The boys swim in 12ft of warm, clear water whilst Paul and Sally go off in the dinghy looking for signs of life. They return saying there were feelings of hostility from the small community they found, so they had set off again to another landing place, where they found a shop and really helpful people. A strange contrast.

" What? *Chase the Lady* again? Just one round and then BED!"

At some hour in the middle of the night, I become aware of a light flashing through the window. On looking out I can see no sign of its cause, and thinking it could be a fishing boat, lay down again. When it happens a second time I get up to investigate meeting Paul in the cockpit, who has also been disturbed. We see a small boat with a very powerful searchlight focused on us by one of two men. This is very scaring until the other man speaks, in fairly good English telling us to pull up the dinghy into the boat as it could get stolen at night by divers and that we are just out of range of their security lights. As this seems to be such a remote, quiet place it is a surprise that there is any security watch at all, or that anyone even knows we are here. It is most disquieting.

At early dawn, Sam looks out and sees a man in a dinghy like ours drifting close in under the cliffs, then of course he can't see ours; panic. Paul and I had managed to haul it up on deck without waking anyone.

That man did look furtive and up to no good though. This is another weird place.

July 13th Misena to Mergellina

At the dawn of another beautiful day, the previous night's fright is soon forgotten and normal water play is resumed until 11.15am, when we sail round the corner to revisit Baia, to show the family the bay of 'dead ships'. Whatever the reason for them, it is a chilling, eerie sight that we are glad to leave.

The sea is now messy with a chop and an irregular swell as we try, not very successfully to sail with head sail only into the marina at Niseda.

As we approach, an officious fancy uniform runs down shouting and waving his arms, *Privato, privato. Militare*! There are no notices to show that this is a NATO base, perhaps they don't want anyone to know.

We back away, wave and look around - it is lunchtime, we are reminded by the two ever-hungry pair. There seems to be plenty of room on the opposite set of pontoons, so we take a chance and just manage to finish a leisurely lunch before being politely told that we cannot stay, "Regatta tomorrow." (I bet!)

Reluctantly, we make our way back to Mergellina, not an exciting prospect but we radio ahead to the *Capitano* and are met and greeted like old friends, then shown into a good position by Louis and his merry men.

Today's outing has only covered 12 miles and adds up to 606miles for the season and 752 altogether from La Ciotat, not exactly breaking any records!

This is the last night of the family holiday, a bit of an anti-climax, particularly as there is not a restaurant near enough for any of us to make the effort to go. We sit back and relax, watching the paraders and the cats looking for rats. "I shouldn't climb on those rocks, Russ. You'll … Oh, dear. The blood has run down onto your clean socks! Fetch the cards. We'll have a round of Chase the lady."

July 14th
This is the last day of their holiday so we must try to make the most of the last few hours. Realising that so far, we have seen very little of Naples itself, we take the bus to Castel Nuovo in the area of Santa Lucia. This imposing castle with its castellated towers and deep moat, was built in 1282 by Charles of Anjou, then rebuilt by Alphonsus 1st of Aragon, but it is closed because it is Sunday. Nearby is the San Carlo Opera House, the Royal Palace and a has-been grand arcade. A service is in progress at the Francesco di Paola Basilica in the Piazza del Plebiscito, hence we only see the outsides of these fine buildings, which all look in need of some attention.

Hot, footsore and over-loaded with culture, we come to a little haven in a public park where we all flop gratefully into swinging seats for cold beers and of course, ice creams for Russ and Tom. The ice creams make them hungry and thirsty again, needing another stop further down the park for lemonade and sandwiches. We don't often have chance to spoil them!

Sally intended to buy some cakes but communication breaks down concerning the thousands of lire and she flees, leaving the puzzled man holding the parcel.

By 4.15pm it is time to catch the airport buses, then say our sad farewells in the departure lounge and agree that it has been a fun–packed two weeks. We are both very subdued this evening. "Isn't it quiet? What, no card games?"

July 15th
How lucky we have been! This morning brings a howling force 7 wind, rain and a mighty thunderstorm, otherwise there is a funereal quietness. No giggling or marauding elephants on deck at dawn.

Mergellina on a wet day is unbelievably grim. The locals appear more miserable than ever and look at you resentfully if you are a visitor or have a boat, but there is the shopping to do to replenish all food, drinks and toilet rolls.

The sun shines weakly in the evening and we try to tidy up, but with an obvious lack of enthusiasm. Being alone again is a great anti-climax after two weeks of high activity, and feels a bit like being convalescent!

July 16th

Although the sun is back, we are still finding it hard to get motivated and don't feel like sailing yet. What shall we do?

Remembering that we have not seen Pompeii, and we are here to see the sights, a sudden burst of action has us running for the bus to Garibaldi station for the Trans-Vesuvian Line, which has a halt almost across the road from the ruins. Admission is free on showing our passports.

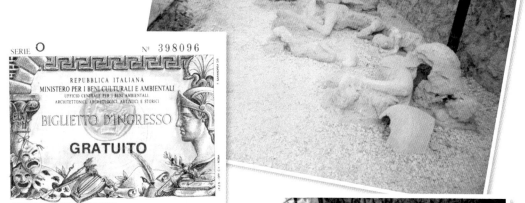

In 80BC the town of Pompeii came under Roman domination and was a favourite resort for rich Romans, many of which settled here. It became a booming town with a port, numerous trades and industries, and a population of over 20,000 inhabitants. In 62AD an earthquake caused extensive damage to the town, but before full restoration was complete, a nearby volcano, Vesuvius erupted in August 79AD. Within two days Pompeii was buried under a layer of cinder, mud and pebbles to a depth of over 20 feet.

Much of the population died instantly when overcome by the volcanic ash and some of the first remains were found in the 17th century, but it was not until 1754 that systematic excavations began.

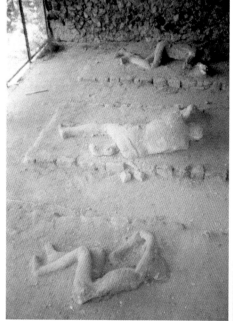

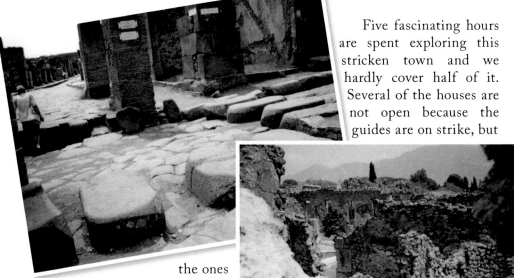

Five fascinating hours are spent exploring this stricken town and we hardly cover half of it. Several of the houses are not open because the guides are on strike, but the ones we do see are in an amazing state of preservation with the wall-paintings fresh and bright, as in Herculaneum, portraying some interesting postures in the bordello. Many houses have descriptive names such as, 'The House of the Golden Cherubs', 'House of the Faun', 'House of the Great Fountain', and 'House of the Tragic Poet' to fire the imagination.

The Stabian Baths have both men's and women's baths with hot, cold and tepid pools, changing rooms, and the under floor heating running between the pools, again as in Herculaneum.

Several well-placed fountains seem to serve as meeting and refreshment places, where you can refill your water bottles. After lunch under shady pine trees, we are ready for a mile or so of chariot-grooved streets, which have stepping stones at cross roads for the purpose of avoiding streams of water after rain, and the garbage brought with it.

Next is the Great Theatre that could hold 5,000 spectators, an *Odeon*, which is a covered theatre to hold about 800 people, (Now we know how the name of some of our cinemas originated.) and barracks for the gladiators. These Romans had a very organised and sophisticated lifestyle even 2,000 years ago.

The museum, or antiquarium, hold the historical records and many distressing mouldings of the animals and humans in the positions in which they had died. All seem to be shielding their faces. Pompeii is a sad place compared with Herculaneum, where most of its population were able to escape.

There is still much more to see but the brain, feet and legs are shouting, "Enough." It is a relief that the railway station is so close but the last stretch back to the boat is demanding. It has been a thought-provoking day.

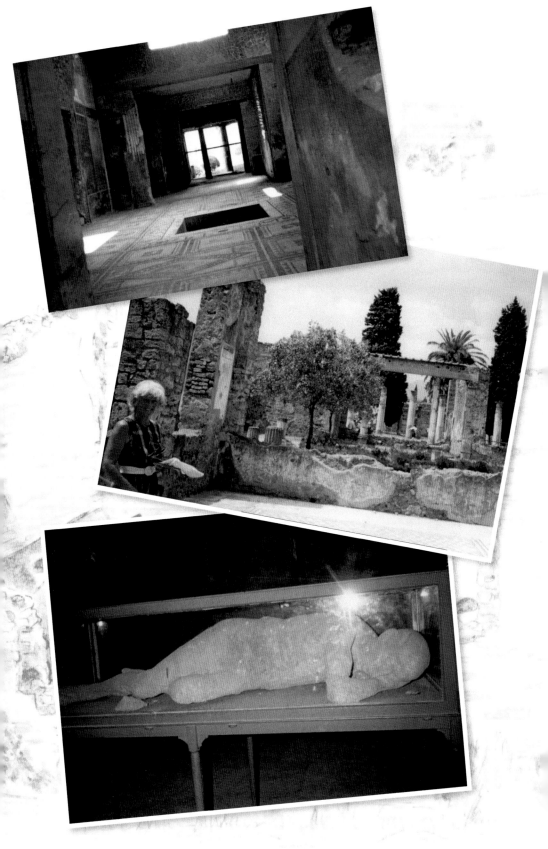

Chapter 5

Sweet and Sour
(assorted morsels)

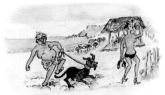

Dog's Body

July 17ᵗʰ Mergellina to Casamicciola

The two weeks with the family have been happy and relaxed, but for some time Sam has felt a bit anxious about our next move, conscious that there always seems to be some snag or hassle in each port that takes away some of the pleasure. He is twitchy and losing weight, yet I would like to carry on, which causes intermittent interludes of slight domestic discord. Are we becoming faint-hearted or are we too old at sixty five for this way of life? Surely not.

It is greatly disappointing to feel that we will not achieve what we set out to and I feel cheated, but Sam will not have his arm twisted. I have tried! So, this is to be the turning point and we sadly must begin our way back. It may be slight consolation to realise that the further down Italy, the further distance it is between ports and the people are poorer, so greater is the resentment of foreigners with a boat - apparently.

Hoping this is a right decision, we agree to enjoy the pleasant places at a much more leisurely pace on our way back.

Now being resigned to Sam's wishes we pay up, visit the bank, replace the gas bottle and leave as quickly as possible before any second thoughts creep in.

An easy 17.5 mile motor sail across to the Isle of Ischia and we return to Casamicciola, because it is familiar and we feel comfortable here. Still feeling somewhat cheated at this upsetting anti-climax, I take myself off for a swim to cool off while Sam has a siesta.

Spirits are lifted, but we are both a bit quiet this evening.

July 18ᵗʰ Casamicciola to Isle of Ponza

With a fidgety mixture of excitement and apprehension of the unknown, we make an early rise to get away. An embarrassing swing across several anchor chains is watched by two smirking security guards as we leave, together with an Italian yacht at 7am. A course of 280^0 is set for the islands of Ventotini and Ponza under mainsail, foresail, and a murky sky. Switching on the autopilot (George), we sit back and relax as we gradually overtake the Italian yacht. This prompts them to crack out the huge mainsail and with a salute and a wave they shoot past.

'George' now becomes temperamental and takes us round in circles, so we have to take turns to helm again. The tip of Ventotini is spotted at 11.15am, the same time as the Italian yacht is seen disappearing over the horizon.

The sun is now over the yardarm, and by the time we have downed a small warm beer, Ponza is vaguely visible in the distance. When two miles off Ventotini, the second beer decrees that we go straight on to Ponza whilst conditions are favourable, even though the sea is a bit confused, it's hot and has been slightly boring for the last ten miles of the 47 in all.

At 3.30pm we are circling round the crowded harbour looking for space when we spot a new empty pontoon near to a dredger and are beckoned in and assisted to moor up. The area is obviously still under construction. There is only one other boat; no one asks for money; there is no office in sight; it can't be free; we don't like to ask.

The little community smacks of toy-town, with yellow, pink and blue box-like houses piled up round the quayside, a yellow cathedral, little white lighthouse and caves in the rocks on the small beaches. A most attractive, quiet scene.

Quiet? In the early evening countless huge power-boats with their uniformed crew, come pouring back from their day time jaunts, into the docks and the bay. Next to us looms 'The Godfather' with his four glamorous daughters and entourage – I think this is going to cost *lotsa lira*. "Ah well."

July 19th

Apart from The Godfather whooping it up until 3am it was a peaceful night. Then comes the shock – for the privilege of a new hosepipe and a bit of planking, 45,000 lira (£22.50) is collected by two 'heavies' at 8.15am, giving rise to much water activity to ensure getting our money's worth by filling up the tanks, laundering and showering under the hose. It is remarkable how long the water stays hot in a hosepipe.

Prices in the few little shops are twice as much as on the mainland and three times English costs. Enquiring at the Harbour Office in hope of a place in the main harbour, we are told that if you are prepared to move every few hours or so, then you can come in. We are not. Also, the wall is too high for easy access and since the walking the plank game, we now have no gangplank.

Rather reluctantly we leave the pontoon to anchor in the bay along with a number of others and hope that the weather stays fair. By dinghy we call on another English yacht and invite them over, and during the wine-induced chat, hear that they are on the way to Greece for the winter. That hit rather a raw spot, and although I managed a pleasant, "Very sensible" at the time, I did have to apologise to Sam later for peevishly pointing out that, "THEY are going to Greece."

The bay fills up in the evening and about thirty boats are swinging round us with dinghies busily ferrying their passengers ashore, stirring up a wash as they go.

Utilising the mizzen halyard and winch makes it so much easier to lower the outboard engine to fix onto the dinghy, which has to be used every time we want to go ashore. Hearing that there is a £5 charge to look after a dinghy, we leave it on another pontoon and just hope it will be there later.

A typical battered old bus rattles us up narrow winding roads round a spectacular coastline right to the end of the island where there is a bar, a viewpoint, two or three little houses and nothing else. The bus stops and waits a few minutes for you to take in the ambience, then drops us off at Le Forna on its return, where the road descends steeply to Cala Fiola. This small inlet is a delightful swimming hole with rocks, caves and surprisingly, a bar of sorts. In reality, this oasis is a weather-beaten shed built into the rocks with two rickety tables and a few chairs teetering on the uneven rocky edge above a twelve-foot drop into the water. "Don't fidget and don't drop anything!" Sitting very still, we patronise it for an excellent ham sandwich and a plastic cup of beer straight from the can. It is right to assume there are no toilet facilities here.

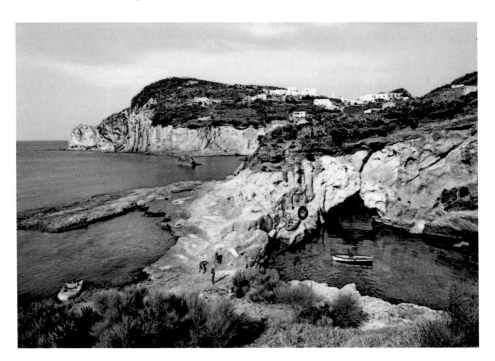

Swimming in the clear turquoise water, we wish we had snorkels or even a towel, yet there is a hosepipe on a stick to serve as a shower for which they enterprisingly charge 75p per shot.

Being the only people waiting at the bus stop, the driver recognises us and we enjoy the lovely ride back into Ponza, to find that the dinghy is still where we left it. Another British yacht from Dartmouth has arrived to socialise and exchange books with, they say they are on their way to Greece. "Did you hear that, Sam?"

Yesterday being Sunday, not a lot happened apart from the arrival of a lovely traditional gaff-rigged boat with a young couple and a dog on board, which had come down the canals through Belgium and France. Amongst all the plastic modern craft here, this boat is so noticeable for its different classic lines.

'A funny thing happened on the way to the bank.' In the dinghy we are just gently approaching the pontoon and in readiness, I am leaning over with the painter, reaching for the iron ring to slot it through for tying up. Perhaps I lean too far. Doing a neat header into the harbour water between the ring and the dredger, I manage to grab my straw hat on the way back up whilst still holding the painter. "I wondered where you had gone," remarked the oblivious spouse.

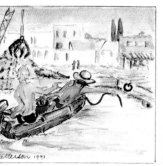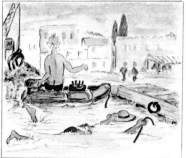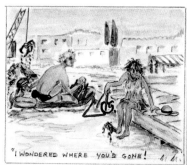

A few squirts from the nearest hosepipe and I am ready to hit the town, although going to the bank and shops with wet hair and a provocatively clinging T-shirt does nothing for ones dignity. It is lucky that my shorts and sandals are in the bag with the returnable bottles, but what the dredger has stirred up is not to be dwelt on as it does not taste too good.

Back on board, fishing is the next project. There are so many fish swimming round the hull. We tempt them with a piece of cheese and catch a pretty seven inch, silver and yellow striped fish but it jumps overboard on the way to the bucket. One that is too small is rehabilitated; the next silver one is easy, but failing to catch another that also gets a reprieve. So much for our supper – pasta again.

Apart from the constant rocking from the wash of the passing craft, it is peaceful at anchor here and at present we have no desire to move on. The daily routine seems to be going ashore in the mornings to the few little shops with the matriarch guarding the door where new bread is fifty pence (1991) for half a brick, and the afternoons are spent swimming, writing or drawing. Sam is deliberating on where to put the deck shower he is installing, and after his fifth interruption when I am trying to design a birthday card for our other grandson's first birthday I am tempted to advise him.

Another attempt at fishing proves futile, as no silver ones come for the cheese, only hundreds of tiny brown ones. We don't enjoy fishing any way.

Glass in hand, the sundown distraction is to watch the antics of the flock of arriving boats trying to get their anchors to hold. On one of them, we greet an American couple in a Moody 30 who are on passage to Sicily. I bite my tongue, smile, "How nice. I hope you have a good trip."

"Let's try a risotto tonight as a change from pasta, and did you notice Sam, I haven't mentioned Greece today."

Next morning ashore, a call at the post office to read the weather forecast shows NW force 7 with thunderstorms, but it never states whether it means – now, later or imminent. Do we stay and hope that the anchor holds, or make a twenty-three mile run back to the mainland? Sam gets twitchy again, a few words are exchanged and a jot of gloom descends, but not for long.

By the time we have walked up to the little lighthouse to gaze at the sea state then back again, Sam is thirsty and the thoughts of moving are soon forgotten. The small bar overlooking the dredger at work has the cheapest tariff yet, obviously the location affects the price.

Next, we enquire the cost to fill up with water. On one pontoon they charge £3 and a few yards further along it is £10, so now we know which one to go to!

Meanwhile, a Moody 36 from Hamble has anchored near us, and so there is much to talk about since that is where we live. An invitation to join us later is gratefully accepted and we learn that they too, are on the way to Greece. And I daren't say a word!

July 26th

The wind starts to moan at early dawn, just softly at first but gradually increases during the day. Fortunately, it is an off-shore wind and the cliffs give some shelter, although the sea is ruffled. So far there is no discomfort.

The post office Meteo board still reads *Forza 7, mare mosso* (rough with thunderstorms). We telephone the family, all are fine, including uncle Fred, and we ask for our mail and new cheque book to be sent to Fumicino.

Walking along some of the back lanes to see as much as possible of this island, we come across some most attractive houses set higgledy-piggledy down the cliffs, each with prolific growths of tomatoes, figs, lemons and apricots, and all just tantalisingly out of reach.

The trip back in the dinghy is frisky and we return very wet to see that the bay is like Piccadilly Circus with boats dragging their anchors motoring round to find a good hold. Many craft, including ourselves think it is advisable to put out a kedge anchor from the stern-to prevent to much swinging. Dinghies are blowing in circles and Sam gets himself a bit wound up in the rope, but he is not alone.

Everyone is standing on the bows anxiously gazing down at their anchor chains and everyone else's too. Then, with a grand flourish in an out sized dinghy, comes the Italian officialdom - a driver, a 'frogman' and a gold-braided, white-

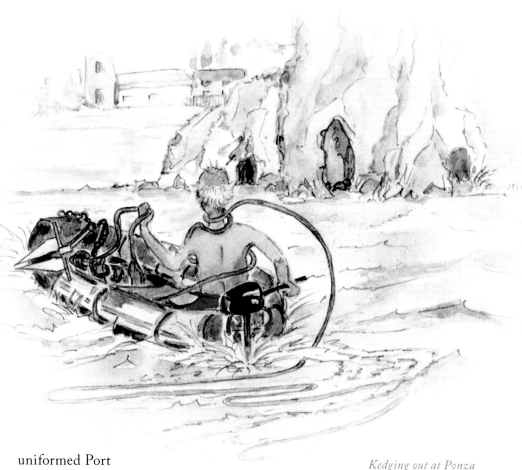

Kedging out at Ponza
"a bit wound up"

uniformed Port
Official, who stands
up to look very important as he
issues megaphoned orders to several boats that they must move closer into
the bay. If the owners are not on board then their anchors are pulled up and
the boat towed further in. What chaos ensues.

We wonder why, what is coming? It is already blowing a force 6.
"Whoops, oh dear," and you can hear the laughter ripple from boat to boat as
the white uniform suddenly tips head first overboard and is dragged back by
the seat of his once pristine, white trousers, still holding his megaphone. He
does not look quite so imposing now.

A few minutes later, the reason for all this to-do becomes apparent. There
is much hooting as the very large ferry arrives, making a much wider swoop
than usual on entering the harbour less than 30 feet away from us. You can
almost see right up the passengers' noses.

A lovely *Swan 50* is having difficulty trying to anchor. I warn Sam not to
laugh when its tenth vain attempt is made, for just as we are about to step into
the dinghy the official swooped up again. "You will move into 20ft depth. Big
ferry comes!" Having seen the previous performance we obey, taking up both
anchors and motor round and round. Anchor here, too close to another boat;

anchor there and the wind blows us off line; next try, too close to the rocks; try again, it doesn't hold. "It serves you right for laughing at the *Swan*."

Another ferry arrives making an even greater arc, and we return to our original place to realise that all we need to have done was to shorten up our chain. Later, we hear that all this rumpus was caused by the ferry captains wishing to make known their protest about the number of boats in the anchorage.

A happy hour or so is spent with the Hamble crew exchanging books, old newspapers, advice and wine as we listen to the wind whining through the rigging.

Since it now seems too much bother to put out the kedge anchor again tonight, a few bearings are taken off the lighthouse and the starboard hand harbour entrance light, just in case we might drag.

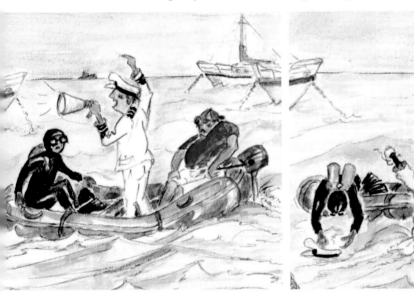

"All boats move to 20' depth. Big ferry comes"

July 27th

With one ear each and an occasional peep, most of the night is spent on 'anchor watch', quite unnecessarily as there was no shift at all. As long as the wind stays away from the east there is shelter. Although the horizon is clear and very blue, there are a few big 'cauliflower' thunderheads lurking. Sam decides to stay so moves closer in, and at the second try is satisfied – I think he is beginning to like anchoring. Very well timed too. The morning ferry comes hurtling in daringly close to the others again. So this is why the harbour authorities are being so neurotic, the ferries are certainly making their protest felt.

With a charming young twosome off a London yacht, we spend an amusing hour watching the shuntings of the new arrivals as they vie for a position to anchor. One sleek yacht succeeds at his sixth attempt, for which the skipper gets a general round of applause and makes a showy bow.

What trivia amuses you when flopping about in the middle of a bay.

July 28th

During the night the wind eases; a sickly rolling takes its place so we abandon our beds for the saloon settees and put up the lee-cloths to prevent us falling onto the floor. Another disturbed night creates two zombies bouncing across in the dinghy to go shopping, which amounts mostly to bottles as the available food on the island is becoming boring – unless you are a pizza or spaghetti addict.

In the market there are great swordfish, tuna and other unknown, fiercely ugly fish, all looking long-time dead and attracting the flies. The meat is unappealing, the long coils of sausages seem mostly made of fat, "Oh, dear. It's chicken breast again. I know what to do with that."

Lugging the bags, we see a tunnel with a sign pointing to Laguna beach, it is quite a long one with its walls showing evidence of Roman times, having the typical diamond-shaped flint stones lining parts of the sides. Eventually the tunnel opens up onto a passable stony beach, its only feature being a shed serving as a bar.

Since the shopping needs a rest, we take refreshment on oily chairs at a dusty table teetering on the stones. For two tins of lager we pay £4 and feel a bit exploited, but they later bring two glasses and a dish of peanuts as a bonus. There is not another soul in sight to provide interest. Strange place.

Two more English boats have arrived. The one nearest is flying the same pennant as our home yacht club and etiquette demands that we should also be flying ours, but after a quick search the crumpled, weather-beaten and faded flag is considered too tatty for display. We invite the two fellow club members to join us later and no sooner had we said, "Cheers," when a smart 40ft local yacht swoops in too fast, then comes to a sudden halt very close to our bows, almost catapulting the posing *bella señorita* head first over the side as the yacht swings onto us. The menfolk are quick to fend it off but the señorita loses her balance and screams her way back to the safety of the cockpit. It is then that Sam notices the cause of the event - the yacht has wound our kedge anchor warp round its keel. Thinking that if we let out some slack the kedge would sink to the bottom and free itself, but the impatient Latin had other ideas. He set his engine hard astern, which zaps the rope through Sam's hands until it comes to the end and he is forced to let go or be dragged overboard. So there, just visible, is our kedge and 100 feet of new line lying on the seabed.

When the astound wears off, positive thinking brings the little grapple anchor into use as we fish for the kedge. At the seventh attempt, with a sigh of relief we hook it up from 23 feet down, just as the two Italians come rowing across to shout, "Excuse me, excuse me, excuse me," and we can reply with, "No problem," which is a phrase every nationality seem to understand.

With that slight diversion over we can settle back to the matters in hand, a half forgotten glass and tale-swapping chatter with the new acquaintances, who say they are on their way to Malta for the winter. 'Button your lips,' I say to myself. Several social engagements occupy the next day, it is becoming like our stay on Elba and is most pleasant. One visit is made to a very young pair who have a beautiful eighteen-month-old daughter with blonde curls and big blue eyes, she has lived on the boat all her life and scrambles around with complete confidence. Returning, the outboard motor begins to cough and splutter, then dies and we have to row back against the force five wind and a choppy sea slopping over bow.

July 30th Ponza to Felice Circio

The wind has turned during the night, bringing a nauseating roll straight into the bay and a few boats have already left. There are two options – either roll all day, perhaps not being able to get ashore or leave despite the sea state in hope of improvement.

At 8.30am both anchors raise easily, bringing up mounds of seaweed that slither across the deck while making ready to go out for a look. The sea is messy yet bearable, with just a light wind as we approach the forbidding rocks off the ends of Ponza and the small island of Zannone. Navigating by tourist maps has its limitations, and we are not sure which gap to pass through. Having got part way through one channel we get cold feet and turn back to where a ferry is seen, so we follow it. Moments later another ferry passes straight through the gap we had shied away from. "Oh, bother!"

Nearer to the mainland, the sea quietens and San Felice marina, where we have been before is entered at 1pm after a fair passage of 21.2 miles, and for once we have no embarrassing manoeuvres when mooring up. This is a pleasant port, having a chandlery, little shops, a bar and a small sandy beach, and most of all, we enjoy the hosepipe opposite the stern.

When going to pay, we optimistically take their last month's receipt hoping they would not charge the summer price. It worked. 21,000 lira is more than enough.

Our mileage from San Remo is now 669.36, and the total from La Ciotat 824.68. I think we may have covered more distance cycling than sailing.

On the next day it is grey with rain driving across in a north-easterly wind, making us very thankful to have left Ponza yesterday. The cockpit drains are very slow again, especially with the rain. Sam disconnects the pipes and now there is a gallon of evil-smelling water in the bilges from which we extract paper, hair, crisps, another beer-bottle top and an unidentifiable, important-looking chromium nut. The outlet has definitely improved now.

Since the *Capitano* has already summed up tomorrow's weather for us in two words, "No good," plans are made to further explore this area on the bikes.

On the next boat is a French skipper who has paralysed legs. He and his wife have very ingeniously adapted ropes and pulleys to enable him to get in and out of his wheelchair from the boat. They are very young and we do so much admire their courage and enthusiasm; they also have a pretty grey and white cat called Pom Pom.

August 1st

A stiff breeze persists and the sea is rough. Not a day for sailing so the little folding bicycles are lifted over the guard-rails, together with swim kit, water-proofs, map and a packed lunch, ready for a day of discovery. On the way to look for a bank in a newer part of town we find a long street of good shops, some fresh rolls and good tomatoes. Once out of the centre, the road is flat and rural, with mountains on the right hand side and woods and fields on the left. After about three and a half miles we reach the duned coast, where the sea is raging onto the shore and the red flags are flying. On a slight rise backing the beach are beautiful villas having a sea view on one side and a long lake on the other.

Chaining the bikes to a 'No parking' sign at the side of a shed-like restaurant, there is a board walk through the dunes to where we join the multitude bathing on the edge of the surf. It is refreshing, exhilarating, and a little dangerous as there is a strong under-tow and no one ventures out very far.

Lunch is taken with a sprinkling of blown sand followed by a *Cornetto*. The caves and Paola's tower on the headland do not seem to be accessible, so we return by a different route through the forest, glimpsing more opulent villas behind their security fences and grand wrought iron gates which display the customary warning *Attenti al cane*.

On return, another play in the surf on the small adjacent beach cannot be resisted, especially as it can be followed by a shower from the warm water in the hosepipe. The cup of tea is nectar as we reflect on the day out, and how much we appreciate being in a safe mooring and not having to worry about the weather, or being told to leave.

August 2nd

There is no mention of moving on today in spite of the favourable conditions, and we convince ourselves that the sea will still be disturbed from yesterday besides, we like it here.

The streets through the new town are attractively lined with alternate pink and red oleander trees in full bloom, and there is no sign of litter or scruffiness. A modern church is a confection of vivid blue tiled, domed roof, a pink and white circular main building with a white bell-tower and a bright blue vicarage, set in a garden of palm trees and bright magenta bougainvillea. In contrast, there is the first supermarket we have seen for a long time and notice the considerable difference in prices compared to the islands.

'Surf's up' on the little beach for a romp in the waves, but at 68°F the water feels a bit cool. Basking, reading, glass in hand as the sun sinks down behind Circes' mountain we can enjoy the elements, since we are not going anywhere tomorrow either. This way of life is not all doom and gloom.

August 3rd

This town seems to be a comparatively new development as a resort, even the back streets are opulent with picturesque villas, perhaps it is where the Romans spend their holidays.

As advised at the marina, we call in at the reception desk of the very modern hotel for information on the locally famous *Guattari* cave, prompting the over-helpful receptionist to go into full flood with a detailed history, and since it happens to be in the hotel garden she organises the gardener to give us a guided tour. This charismatic old chap with twinkling eyes, burbles away happily in Italian for half an hour, with just an occasional English word here and there. We manage to work out that in 1939 the rocks in that part of the garden were blasted out because they had become unsafe, and as a result the cave was exposed containing the skull of a Neanderthal man who had lived about 60,000 years ago. Our guide enthuses over the many fossilised animal bones he proudly shows us; *originale* he assures. Our modest tip seems to delight him also.

Playtime on the beach today is cut short by the arrival of a large cauliflower cloud bringing a spectacular thunderstorm. Moving on tomorrow is hinted at, but shelved in favour of another leisurely day here.

August 5th San Felice to Nettuno

Both wake early and already, Sam is chewing himself up again because we are letting go of the wall. Out of the harbour at 7.15am into a hazy, oily calm sea with not a puff of wind and needing the motor on for all the twenty five miles. On rounding the Circeo headland we see all the renowned five caves and Paola's tower again before traversing the long, flat, dune-backed bay. The only excitement is from the two fast customs and excise launches zooming past to over take and halt a large luxury power boat, which is then joined by a police boat. Quite a to-do, but we never found out why.

In good time for lunch, we arrive in the stark, new, concrete marina at Nettuno where we visited briefly in June and moaned about the pontoons being too high again, making access like an assault course. Obviously, these marinas are not built with small yachts in mind.

Looking at the town, it is an odd mixture of medieval ramparts and ugly blocks of flats, but then we find out that much of it was destroyed by the allied landings in 1944-5, and was hastily and cheaply rebuilt. However, it seems to have adequate, handy supermarkets and useful shops.

An English boat *Dabber* has arrived next to us from Poole, so Roy and Tina are invited across for a happy hour when the usual experience-swapping session ensues. If we think we have had a few problems, they are trivial compared to theirs. Their gear-box is dead and must return home when they have found someone to repair it. They have very little money and now their gas has run out.

August 6th

Tina tells us where to find the market, and more time than anticipated is taken browsing through the colourful stalls of fresh fruit and vegetables, cheeses, yards of coiled sausage and food we haven't seen for weeks. The prices are much more realistic too.

An hour on the beach is enough for today, before hauling the bikes up off the stern-to go exploring and look at a newish Basilica, a neglected park and the American War Cemetery, for which we are ten minutes too late as it has just closed.

Tonight we take wine on *Dabber*, commiserating with them whilst watching the local lads who come here to dive off the pontoon. There are fifteen of them between twelve and sixteen years old diving, hanging onto boats, climbing out up the ropes, and becoming a noisy nuisance. They are duly, very loudly reprimanded by the *Capitano,* and a credit to them that they did not answer back and obeyed by keeping away from the boats from then on.

August 7th

By using our ship's telephone via Radio Geneva, it is now possible to send belated birthday greetings to son Paul and also hear that he has posted mail to Fiumicino, and that the friend who wished to come to Brindisi in September, now wants to come and see us near Rome instead.

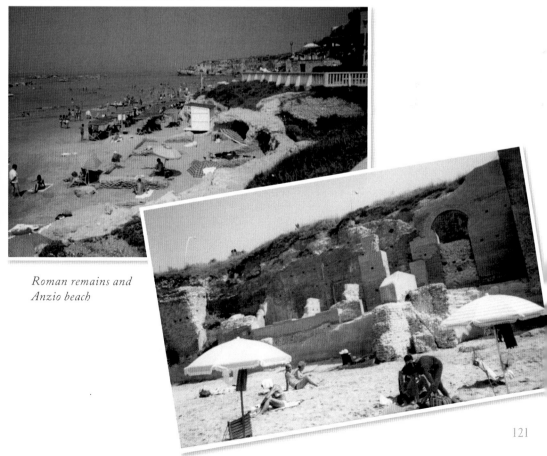

Roman remains and Anzio beach

Although it is always very nice to have company, it is always a problem to be in a suitable place at the right time. Fuimicino is the nearest port for Rome airport but there is no desire to spend nearly six weeks there again, and this marina is too expensive for any length of time.

Since Anzio is the next nearest place, we set off early to cycle there to inspect it. An easy flat ride, only two or three miles away, although we have to push a way through the weekly market on the cliff top, an avenue of cheap shoes, 'designer' sun glasses, watches and the belts with rusty buckles, and no fresh produce. Below is the beach and the remains of one of Nero's palaces, backed by more unknown excavations, and further along is the old Roman harbour.

Quite by chance, we are surprised to meet Roy and Tina. They are trying to find a shipyard to handle their gear-box repairs and as she speaks good Italian, she also manages to wheedle a berth for us - for a month if necessary. We feel a bit easier about that, even if it is not the most picturesque of ports.

For afternoon diversion, we go to find the English war cemetery, just outside Anzio.

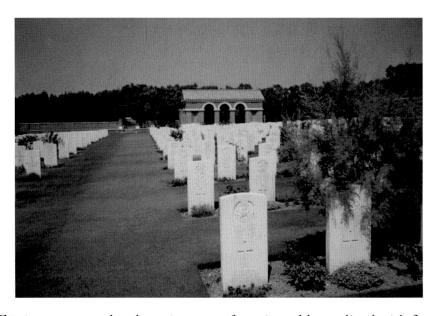

This is a serene, sad and moving area of manicured lawns lined with flowers, and the military precise rows of white gravestones. Each stone, 1,056 in all, has the insignia of the appropriate regiment carved on it together with a chilling inscription that blurs the eyes.

Along with other regiments were the Royal Engineers and Sherwood Foresters who lost so many young lads of 17, 18 and19 years old, and others mainly between 22 and 38 years - all so young, so sad, yet not forgotten or neglected. With regret, we cannot not sign the visitors' book as we have no pen and do not like to ask the two policemen who are patrolling the gates and pointing machine guns at us. For some unknown reason they are stopping traffic with an outsize 'lollipop'. Is it for us to cross the road with the bikes?

After a quick swim, we need to replenish the aperitif fodder as we have asked Roy and Tina over to try and cheer them up. It is now arranged that tomorrow we will ferry them round to Anzio to make another attempt to find a marine engineer.

The local lads are diving here again but are now being very well behaved.

August 8th Nettuno to Anzio

The visitors arrive at 8.40am and since we are not making a meaningful passage, we take the time to waft the two and a half miles in a gentle breeze under the foresail only. Why isn't it like this when we need a long passage?

We moor up in the marina then as instructed, we all shout many times, as loud as we can, "*ALFREDO*", until Alfredo saunters into sight and says we can stay in this berth for a few days until another is available.

Sam makes a start on his job list, but after messily applying anti-foul paint onto a small bung of the depth-finder log, sited under the bunk, he goes back to his book until lunchtime. An afternoon swim has now become routine, but here you have to thread a way through the rows of umbrellas that shield the glistening brown bodies sprawled across their loungers. The sea is warm but the stirred up sand spoils its clarity.

It looks as if we shall have to stay here for about five weeks. We don't want to back track or arrive in Fuimicino too soon, and Elba is over a hundred miles away, so we must just get to like it here.

There are the antics of the children's dinghy class to watch and there has been a noisy football commentary for the last three hours, but we are not complaining as we are well sheltered from the open sea and it is not expensive.

August 9th

Cycling round the local shops we hope to find something different for the bored taste buds, such as real bacon, gammon steaks or pork chops. Alas no, the choice is still between which shape of pasta you prefer, which is the best designed label on the rows of tinned tomatoes and what type of bread you want to build your fortress. With fresh fish I am squeamish, recoiling from the smell and the reproachful look in their eyes; I prefer it in batter from the chippy.

Sam does the second job on his list and paints another two inches of the impeller before succumbing to the effects of a small lunchtime beer.

Alfredo asks us to move to another berth, which is handy for the hosepipe but opposite the coffee bar where a crackling tape recording is tearing the heart out of some love sick lothario. When 'mama and papa' see our British ensign they change the tape to renderings of *Lilli Marlene* and *Roll out the Barrel*. Leaving Sam with his job list, I take the empty wine bottle to the 'cave', where it is refilled, petrol pump fashion from huge tanks. At roughly £1.15 for one and a half litres, I am assured by the proprietor that it is *Bellissimo* - and so it should be.

Lilli Marlene greets my return; it sounds like the original Marlene Dietrich recording. Tina and Roy come over for the last time as tomorrow they are flying home. We promise to pump out their leaking bilges occasionally.

By 10pm the Piano Bar on the promenade is in full fortissimo jangle.

August 11ᵗʰ

The church bells are chiming out the same cracked little tune as in Ponza and this calm and peaceful day really feels like Sunday. There are posters flapping on the lampposts advertising an orchestral concert, so we take a leisurely stroll along the beach towards the white domed confection of the arts centre to enquire about obtaining tickets. From a hundred yards away we can hear a rehearsal in full blast, no-one seems to notice as we gradually filter up into the balcony seats to enjoy over an hour of energetically conducted classical favourites performed by the Symphony Orchestra of Bulgaria! How do you follow that unexpected pleasure? With a cold *birra alla spina* (beer from the tap), from one of the many beach bars – just one, and make it last.

Further along the promenade an open air art exhibition of local talent is not too impressive, but the timing of *Lilli Marlene*, as we step back on board is certainly worthy of attention. Lunch is accompanied by the *Beer barrel polka*, Vera Lynn's *White Cliffs of Dover* and other war time oldies. For the next month we are to hear this same crackling recording about eight times a day – perhaps it is meant to be a friendly gesture, or are they poking fun at us?

Having now decided to sit it out here until it is time to collect our friend, the days pass pleasantly with domestic chores, replacing the teak deck plugs and a daily beach session, for which we now go to the other side of the marina where the water is much clearer. This beach is the one with the added interest of Nero's villa. He was born in Anzio, which was then called Antium and he reigned from 54–68AD. We wonder if he and Caligula built sandcastles on the beach as children, unlike many of today's Italian children we observe.

To check if there is any mail, a visit to Fiumicino takes almost all day involving a rickety bus ride through pines, farms, market gardens, and gently rolling terrain to Rome, then five stops on the Metro and a train to Fiumicino. The post office is reached just on its point of closing. There are four letters but not the cheque book we are becoming anxious for; it is our only means of getting money without the cards. In the absence of any pleasing lunch bars, we buy a sandwich and enjoy reading the letters sitting on the canal bank amidst the ants until time to face the return on local transport. It is noticeable that the fields have lost the greenness, and now look brown and parched.

Lilli is underneath the lamplight waiting to greet us back, and being tired and thirsty, *Roll out the Barrel*!

As promised, we pump out Roy's bilges as it is not too far to walk along the beach into Nettuno, and it gives us the opportunity to browse round the chandlery for items they don't seem to stock elsewhere. The three same sized jubilee clips that we need are all differently priced, and the attempt to clarify this variation seems to cause a heated argument between the man and wife, although you can never be sure as everyone here sounds as if they are shouting at each other.

The heat and humidity is creating a glut of home made cream cheese, as even the small half litre box of UHT milk barely lasts all day in our ailing refrigerator. Thinking that powdered milk might be a solution, we are sent from the *Alimentari* to the *Pharmacie* and *Drogarie* without success. What, cream cheese again? Mosquitos are becoming a nightly nuisance and are not deterred by the lighted coils, so we have our exercise mozzie bashing in a smoky cabin to the strains of *Lilli* three times nightly!

On the morning of the night we intend to dress up for the next orchestral concert, enthusiasm wanes at the thought of digging under the bunks for a creased, semi posh frock and having to walk a mile in smarter shoes. Instead, we turn up wearing shorts and flip-flops in time for the morning rehearsal again. Wagner's *Tristan and Isolde*, and Tchaikovsky's *Romeo and Juliet* are fervently rendered by the same Bulgarians. During the interval, the elderly double bass player comes across to chat to us about their travels and very seriously adds, "We are not very important, but we are cheap. That is why they like us here."

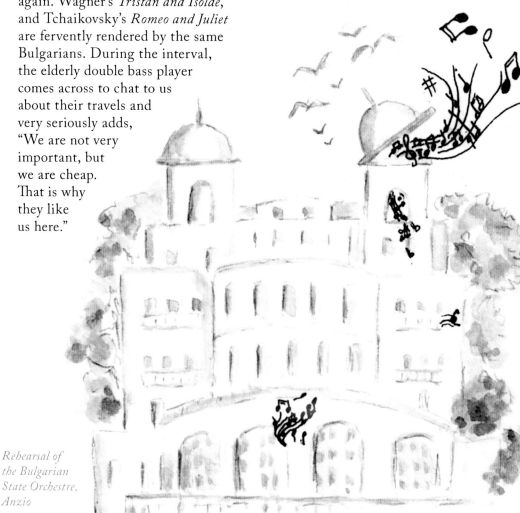

Rehearsal of the Bulgarian State Orchestre, Anzio

Afterwards, a reviving beer at the yacht club costs only 75 pence including service i.e. the bent old waiter pours it from can to glass at your table. Mama and papa spot our approach and here comes *Lilli* again.

Next on Sam's job list is clean out the water tanks - that is when I am conned with his usual devious ploy, "Your hands are smaller than mine." Before long we have the system in pieces and I am up to the shoulders inside with sponges on lengths of wire and my new pop socks for a nylon filter, prior to refilling with fresh water to the sounds of the *Beer barrel polka*.

Mail is still causing anxiety. Paula, the girl in the post office helps us to ring the Fiumicio office to save the palaver of the transport to go there in person, but language problems arise and they think we are wanting to sail there to post a letter.

More futile visits are made, then another clerk fetches Daniella from behind the scenes who speaks passable English and within minutes she has faxed the Fiumicino office with instructions to redirect any mail to Anzio. Two days later we gratefully receive the new cheque book, which was posted three weeks ago. It must have been on a world tour.

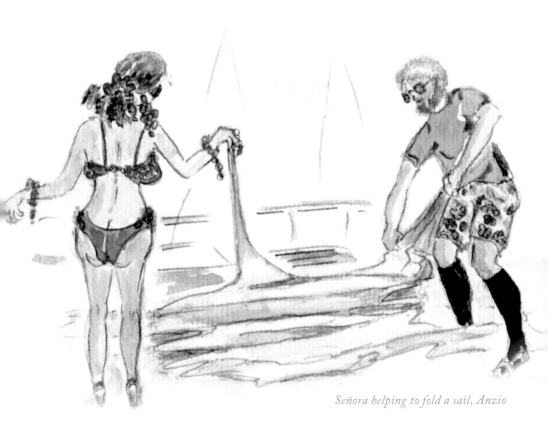

Señora helping to fold a sail, Anzio

On the next boat, a buxom señora, resplendent in a bright blue, crushed velvet, bikini that is festooned with gold braid and pearls, extends a delicate thumb and forefinger to help fold up a sail. This scene distracts me from the sketch of the café family I am trying to capture while 'dad' is sitting in the corner in his vest, with finger poised to press the button on *Lilli*. The three *ormeggiatoris* spend more time at that same table than they do tending the marina.

Not before time, I pluck up courage to go to the hairdresser as my hair is back to the length at which I normally have a haircut. In my absence, Sam has put a few patches on the foresail, replaced the tell tale ribbons that lie flat on the sail when it is set correctly and re-taped the shrouds; that is the extent of today's work.

When we return from the beach there is a space where *Kalivala* should be. The three *ormis* are just moving it further along the quay; now we cannot see the happenings at the café, but can still hear its customary tunes. This same evening we become aware of some splashing sounds coming from between the boats. It does make one curious as to how a blue budgerigar comes to be frantically doing the backstroke among the ropes and no one is looking for it. By the time we reach it with the fishing net, he has breathed his last breath. Mouth to beak resuscitation and heart massage are alas, to no avail.

One hot, steamy morning Sam gives up on buffing up the spinnaker pole, which is showing signs of corrosion after two years without use, instead we walk into Nettuno, pump Dabber's bilges again, then visit the small museum of the Allied Landings. This is mainly taken up with harrowing photographs of the extensive damage to both Nettuno and Anzio, where many buildings can be recognised amongst the tragic mess. The curator tells us of the evacuation of the inhabitants and the severe punishments by the Germans for being caught in town without an official pass. Other memorabilia consists mostly of American souvenirs which have been donated by the local people. The curator is a bit upset they had to refuse a Jeep due to lack of space. Although neither of these towns are truly pretty at this time, it does make you realise the hardships they must have endured and the remarkable recovery they have since made.

On the way back there is time to check out the yacht club, but there are still no other customers just the bent old waiter, which is a shame as it is a pleasant little clubhouse.

A day's weather can almost be predicted by the beach umbrellas – if they are open it is good, if closed then the boats are rolling round in the wind and surge, the surf stirs up the sand and the beaches are deserted. This is when we can enjoy a brisk walk in the fresher air. An English lady with her Italian husband stops to talk, so we ask them back for a cup of tea. They stay on for a G&T then as they leave, extend an invitation to supper and also directions to a spring where the waters are supposed to be very good for you. I did intend to fetch some the next day but we are side tracked by the attentions of a Customs Official who tries to convince us that we are not allowed to stay here, and must go into the other harbour. Having experienced exposed harbours before, I spin him a very pitiful sob story about how his fellow countrymen have robbed us, forcing us to wait for documents and replacement cards. It worked! He obviously now feels guilty enough and gradually relents, but so that his rank is not totally undermined, he reminds us of the *Constituto* that says we must leave Italy within six months. Now he has projected his officialdom, he is happy enough to shake hands.

On the day of the invitation to dinner with the new found friends, Rose and Steph, Sam decides to take out the failing fridge yet again to try and fix the slipping spindle. That done, the new hot water tank is set in position ready for connecting up sometime. Meanwhile, I remember about the spring and take two bottles to fill – we are now awaiting magical results.

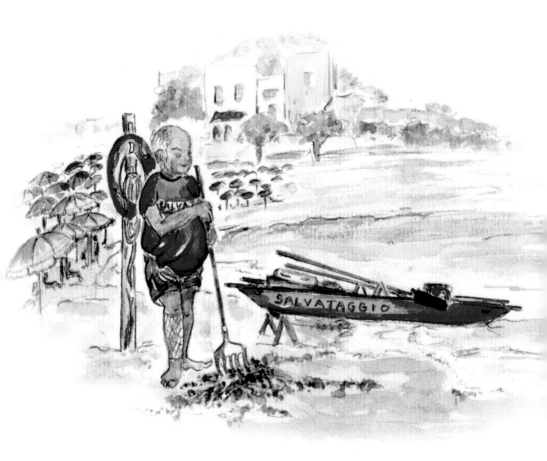

Baywatch! Salvataggio ready for any emergency, Anzio

Steph takes Sam and the afflicted fridge motor to two 'experts' for advice, but they receive the same shake of the head and a shrug. Then we begin making an all out effort to spruce up using the newly installed cockpit shower. We have to hang our clothes on the boom to de-crease as the plug on the iron does not fit here, and neither do the ones for the hair drier or hot brush.

At six o'clock we are picked up by car and taken to Rose and Sam's attractive little house overlooking the bay. The mood is convivial as if we have known them for years instead of just a few days, and Rose is delighted to be able to speak in English for a change. She serves tortellini in cream, chicken with ratatouille, and a lemon meringue pie then, for the first time we sample Grappa, a liqueur that 'graps' you by the throat, warms you up and is advisable only in small doses. How enjoyable it is to have a meal cooked for us and not be rocking about on a boat. Sam is able to mend a clock for them as a return gesture before being driven back clutching a tape recording of *Phantom of the Opera* and a handful of soya beans. We have invited them back for dinner next week.

So far, after repeated draughts of the magical spring water the only noticeable difference is that it is a diuretic and not in the least rejuvenating.

Now being well known at the post office, we only need to look through the door and they shake their head, so we telephone Paul who tells us that uncle Fred has had another bout of bronchitis and, 'Where is his niece when he needs her?' Another guilty phone call hears that he is fit, chirpy and wanting me home.

Anzio is beginning to have that end of season feel, a bit like when the shop shutters slam down at 12.30pm. The beach bars are stacking away some of their deckchairs and umbrellas, and the weather alternates between perfect and unsettled with rough seas.

One hot day there is a surprise invitation from a neighbouring yacht to go for a leisurely sail round the bay, with a heave-to to enjoy a swim in the lovely warm turquoise water. To have a sail at someone else's responsibility just for the fun of it is a rare treat, as is the Grappa we sank on the way back.

The time is approaching when we must think of leaving Anzio so make the most the intermittent good days.

On the day of our dinner party I am frantically flicking through the cookery book only to find that most of the fool proof recipes possible on a boat cooker contain at least one unobtainable ingredient –so keep it simple. One very good custom in both France and Italy is that all the little shops are open on Sunday mornings, so I set off to buy some pork – but come back with chicken. From the café I buy some ice, which is turning to water faster than it can be packed into the fridge, which is now no more than a warm cool box. Fruit, onions and mushrooms are all chopped in a very limited space and out of chaos a palatable meal materialises, albeit not the original menu. We have avocado salad, substituting eggs for unavailable avocados, Pork Orientale, made with chicken, and a spirited fruit salad, all to be helped along with a cheeky, frivolous, nay outrageous local wine at 75 pence per litre. No complaints.

September 9th

The weather gremlins must know we are hoping to leave for Fiumicino tomorrow, making the heavy swell pile relentlessly into the marina, rocking the boats all night, yet the sun shines weakly. Preparations are being made, we pay up, water up and replenish the magical spring water, which so far has had only an adverse effect on the bladder, with no noticeable rejuvenation.

As we bid farewell to Rose and Steph, they tell us that on reaching Fiumicino we must ask for Cigale – a big guy with a fat belly - and he might be able to find a space for us in the yacht basin instead of up the river against the slimy wall.

Then we start to fidget about tomorrow to the familiar tunes in triplicate, from the café. Perhaps we shall miss it.

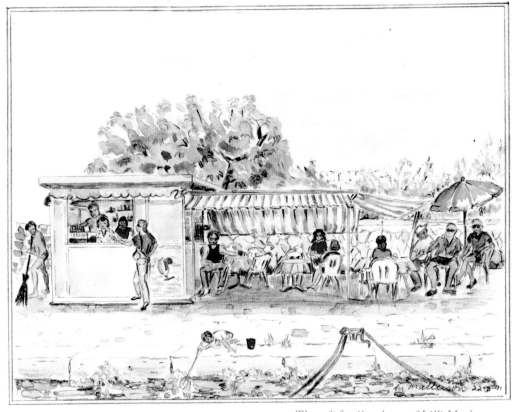

The café family – home of Lilli Marlene

September 10th Anzio to Fiumicino

Sam is fretting about today's passage. "It's barely 29 miles, dear. Don't worry!" Mama and her daughter look most surprised when I take them two little dishes I made from shells as a parting gift. They manage a shy smile, Papa shakes hands, Alfredo helps with the lines and we gently motor out of the marina to music. Guess what?

As usual, the sea state is either all or nowt. It's nowt but a flat glassy calm with no wind, so needing to motor sail along the coast past cliffs, pine trees, and duned beaches until a breeze pipes up from every point of the compass and we need to pay more attention.

You can tell when you are getting close to this port by the murky colour of the water and the amount and variety of debris floating past including tree trunks, plastic bottles and beer cans. At the entrance lies a dredger that did not make very good judgement over the sandbank and is half sunk, on its side being pumped out. No wonder we sometimes get twitchy.

The current runs very fast at the river entrance, so we make aim for the tilting rusty barge which serves as a temporary mooring. It takes two bold thrusts at it before it is near enough to leap across and tie up quickly.

At the Co-operative Harbour Office, our enquiries are met with a curt, "Come back tomorrow." Now what do we do? And there is a man near our boat. It happens that he is just admiring it, and while talking to him we mention about a mooring, and he suddenly points saying, "That's the man you need to see." He does have a certain portliness hanging over the top of his shorts, so I smile and make the approach, "Cigale?"

In less than an hour he has found us a berth inside the crowded yacht basin, although it is a tight squeeze and hanging fourth boat out as they lie bow to stern from the dock. At least we can relax for a few days. Fine until just after midnight when heavy footsteps clomp across the deck to the alongside boat, the engine is run for fifteen minutes and he clomps back again.

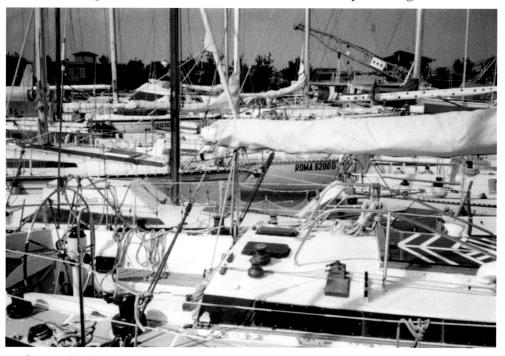

Congested harbour

September 11th

The bicycles would be very useful for rediscovering this town, but the obstacle course over the stays and guard rails of three other boats is tedious enough without any added handicap. A stop at the post office yields nothing, so long overdue Sam braves the barber's chair at the same place as before, and as this is the second time in nearly three and a half months he classes himself as a regular customer.

Contact is made with a refrigerator engineer, Senor Catoni who says he will come to look at it at 9am tomorrow.

The Australian couple that we met last time are still here with engine problems, and we realise that we really have much to be thankful for. The dredger is now looking normal upright against the wall, having been previously so over loaded it caused a serious list and was not aground as thought.

In Anzio there had been no English cruising yachts to talk to, but here seems to be a popular stop over. A young couple row over after anchoring their 34ft *Moody* from West Mersea, they are moving south to Malta and Greece. Somehow, I am losing the inclination to make snide comments – could it be that it is more reassuring to be back in familiar waters and not having to worry about the unknown?

September 12th

Senor Catoni turns up at 11am, takes a brief look at the fridge, scratches his head, shrugs and goes away telling Sam to come to his workshop at 3pm, which he does and it is all locked up. Returning at 4pm all that he can offer is far too expensive to consider, so once again all the happy thoughts of solid butter, fresh milk and cold drinks fade away .

There is a shout across the boats and Mick, from an English motor boat introduces himself with an offer to be taken into Rome tomorrow in his car. That sounds a nice change, although we are not sure what we want to see next. A first rate thunderstorm blows in on a force six wind just before midnight, making all the boats creak and groan, and the rain finds its way in through the hatch right over Sam's head making another entry for his job list.

September13th (Friday)

Although the outlook for today is unsettled, Mick shouts across again and we agree to go and find Tivoli instead of Rome. We pack ourselves into a very small Fiat car, me sharing the back seat with a large black Labrador dog with halitosis, all its blankets, chewed toys and neglected bones. After an hour on motorway and ring road there are directions to Villa Adriani (Hadrian's Villa), so that is the first stop.

Built between 125 and 134AD, it seems to be more of a whole town than just a villa. There are baths, libraries, theatres, barracks, temples, gardens and even a hospital with well preserved mosaic floors in the wards. Being so extensive, we get lost a few times and are put back on course by an American family

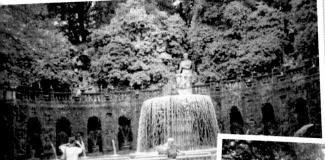

with a proper guidebook. A model on display depicts the original concept, which is very beautiful and almost looks modern.

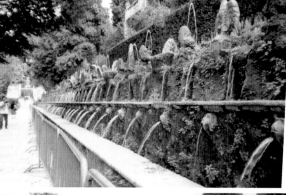

Next we come to Villa d'Este. A complete contrast, being built in 1550 on the site of an old Benedictine monastery. It is entered by way of the original cloisters into rooms almost devoid of furniture, but which have ornate Renaissance paintings on the walls and ceilings. The main attraction here are the famous gardens and incredibly ornate fountains. One is sculpted by Bernini another is akin to a three story building, with organ sounds created by the flowing water. Then we come to the amazing avenue of a hundred fountains where it is so peaceful

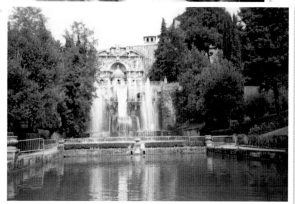

under the pine and Cyprus trees. On a terrace overlooking the gardens and countryside beyond, is an incongruous snack bar offering hefty, boring, pricey sandwiches – the dog fared well!

Wandering twice round the back streets of Tivoli we notice Villa Gregoriana, which also looks interesting. However, we pass it by thinking there is not enough time but are then surprised by a magnificent view across numerous high waterfalls cascading down the mountainside into the river Aniene.

The idea of returning via the Appian Way is thwarted by policemen, one way streets and becoming snarled up in the rush hour traffic - despite having a map. By the time the Colosseum is spotted, signs for Fuimicino appear so we miss the Appian Way.

Arriving back tired and in a heavy downpour and thunderstorm, we are most grateful that the rain held off for this interesting day, as sitting next to a muddy wet dog with halitosis would not have been joyful!

Public Baths

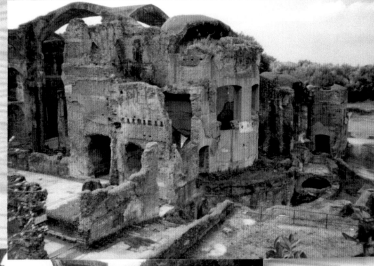

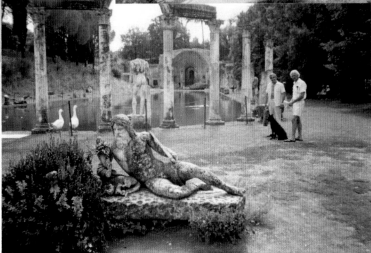

Mike & Sam with Negrita the dog who gave Sam his cold

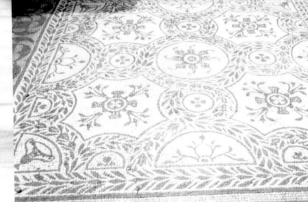

Mosaic floor in hospital ward

September 14th

More thunderstorms. Sam swaps a car compass, which is not very functional, with Mick's hand held fluorescent lamp which is not much good either. We decline another offer of a ride into Rome on account of feet still suffering from yesterday's trip. Sam is in full flood with a cold that he says he caught from the dog, and I must stay within dashing distance of the boat having recklessly indulged in beer, salad and figs at lunchtime.

Between deluges we manage to dry some laundry, lug two five gallon drums of diesel oil across the four decks to fill up the fuel tank, and also drag yards and yards of hosepipe across for the water tank. We should nearly be ready to receive our guest.

The outing we turned down, a visit to the museum of Roman Galleys Mick said was not as good as expected and it had rained, so we have not missed anything.

September 17th

The weather has a more settled feel and from early morning there is much activity with boats being shuffled around in the basin, making our access to the dock even more of an obstacle course than ever when we decide to go last minute shopping, call at the bank and give the dog a bone.

Our anxiously awaited temporary crewman, Des arrives at mid day bearing letters, magazines, gifts in bottles and so much news – it feels like Christmas! After a drink at a forgettable canal side bar and a lazy lunch, torpor sets in and sailing is postponed until tomorrow.

In search of the fleshpots of Fuimicino after supper, we take a nightcap in the same grotty pavement bar amid the cigarette ends and flea ridden cats. The men stick to beer while I grapple with a Grappa, then even before the last sip the shutters are slammed down on the bar and the chairs and tables are almost taken from under us. One may wonder why we did not patronise a better place – we couldn't find one! The alarm clock is set for 5.30am.

September 18th Fiumicino to Cala Galera

At 5.30am it is a surprise to realise that it is still dark at that time and Venus is still brightly shining as we shake ourselves into action and begin to take off the many warps which are tied to three different boats. By this time it is just light enough to push them aside and see the way out of the harbour into the canal, then out into a calm sea. There is not much wind yet, so we have to motor sail half of the way across the long featureless bay with the mountains in the background. The breeze pipes up later, giving a perfect sail on a broad reach for almost thirty miles, even though the sea was slightly rough.

Thinking that we have spotted the island of Giglio through the mist, we steer for the gap between it and the mainland. Whoops! The gap reveals itself to be Cap Ercole, which is on the end of a spit of very flat land and we are aiming to sail through the middle of it. Making an adjustment to port, we then lose the wind and have to motor for the last few miles along the now more rugged coastline to revisit the marina at Cala Galera.

For us, 60.4 miles is a very good day's passage and we had promised ourselves to go out for a meal afterwards but, 'end of season' is here and the nearby restaurants are closed, causing panic in the galley. Supper on board turns out to be an innovative concoction of eggs, cheese, tinned tuna, breadcrumbs and a sauce; it does not have a name but it is surprisingly tasty.

The overall mileage is now 939 nautical miles.

September 19th Cala Galera to Porto Azzuro, Isle of Elba

Des is being helpful but discovers too late that he is topping up the tank from the tap labelled *Non-potabile* - it is OK for scrubbing decks but suspect for drinking. The error is overcome by adding a teaspoonful of embalming fluid (steriliser), in hopes of killing off any evil bugs that may have slipped in. Of course, to be correct we should have emptied the tank, flushed it out and refilled, but that is time consuming and tedious.

The only bit of breeze is on the nose as we leave the marina at 9.15am to motor along, passing spectacular high rocky cliffs, and sighting the islands of Genutri and the real Giglio. Sam thinks he discerns Elba with his bionic eye an hour before anyone else.

Soon afterwards, a red light comes on and an alarm sounds for the water pump, – the engine is over heating. Stopping for investigation, no apparent reason is found so we fan it with last week's *Daily Mail* and, hey presto the red light goes off and we proceed with caution for the last five miles.

Later than anticipated we arrive onto new pontoons in Porto Azzuro at 6.40pm, making happy hour rather delayed but no less happy, before wandering round the little town, which seems to specialise in semi precious stones.

On the water front, a waft from the kitchens of a pizzeria lures us in for supper, which is helped down with a jug of local brew and a toast to an agreeable day.

September 20th Port Azzuro to Porto Ferraio, Elba

The morning is dismal and over cast as we browse in search of a few basic provisions but become side tracked by the fascinating gem shops and give in to a necklace of Hemetite, a local ore, said to only be found on Elba.

After leaving the fuel dock, calculations show that we have been short changed by about £5, so do a hasty about turn back to retrieve it.

As Ferraio is only about sixteen miles along the coast, plans are made to anchor for lunch on the way but somehow, our *Loran* navigator fails to tell us when we had arrived, and the next cove is not at all scenic being opposite to where the Emenite is being mined. In due course an agreeable inlet is reached where the anchor is dropped into thirteen feet of crystal clear swimming water, just off a little bay where the fellas can enjoy the nubile, bronzed scenery that is spread provocatively across the beach.

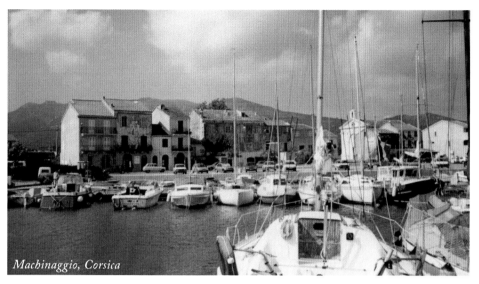

Machinaggio, Corsica

The afternoon breeze blows the boat a bit close to the shore and the depth finder reading shows that there are only four inches of water under the keel. Time to go. With just the big cruising chute sail, we enjoy a leisurely drift round into Ferraio harbour for the second time in three months. We are a bit too late to know whether the old dad had been put out to air on his balcony today.

There are no other cruising boats here now, although a large flashy power boat swoops in next to us, causing a splatter and making a performance out of tying up. *Señora* then puts out a pot of faded dried flowers in the cockpit as a salute to their arrival and her finesse.

September 21ˢᵗ Porto Ferraio to Macinaggio, Corsica

This town wakes up early. Consequently, under cover of heavy black clouds we are ready to leave at 7.45am eating breakfast under sail. There is not much wind yet but by mid day the sun is out, and the once calm sea has become a queasy swell in a fickle wind shift, which spills the beer and rolls the olives across the table.

The afternoon breeze becomes a force five and the waves are higher, giving an exhilarating sail for the forty three miles to the next port.

Mooring up proves a bit tricky, as we blow broadside onto the dock and need much shoving and heaving before succeeding to manoeuvre into a suitable slot at 4.30pm. Now to the hit town.

There is not much of a town to hit, yet it has all the necessary shops and a supermarket stocking pâté and other goodies not seen for a long time, so we make a second trip for further indulgences.

Supper is a little delayed due to Des's testing of an untried Swedish meatball recipe, but no one is heard complaining. On a nearby boat a crowd of happy Germans sing and laugh their way through the night!

The Germans stopped laughing at 5am.

This is a friendly *Capitainerie* with good hot showers, fresh bread and croissants in time for breakfast. Post cards are sent, phone calls made, then we enjoy a beer on the harbour side and the general atmosphere already feels different - more relaxed and comfortable – or is that the beer?

Casting off at 12.15pm the sails are set for the frisky breeze, which is kicking up white horses along the course plotted for Menton on the mainland of France. *Kalivala* creams along, heeling well at an exhilarating pace, until we reach beyond the northern most tip of Corsica. The wind then dies and the sea becomes oily calm, so we take the opportunity to serve up bowls of hearty dog's dinner soup.

Just as we are enjoying this, the autopilot starts being temperamental and won't hold its course, until it has been cursed, threatened and finally, a good thump cures it.

By 5pm, the wind begins to increase knot by knot from 0 to 32knots and the waves gradually build up to what feel to be house sized, and coming broad side on, which is not at all pleasant!

The main sail is dropped and the flapping folds are fought into disorderly submission and tied with one hand, whilst clinging onto the boom with the other. An in-mast or furling main would have been welcome but it is early days yet for that innovation. Having also reduced the fore sail to triangular bandage-size at dusk, we are now ploughing along at seven and a half knots with just the mizzen and fore sail floodlit by the moon on one side and a with grand display of lightning on the other.

We are silent, apprehensive, dry-mouthed and a bit frightened when we change watches every two hours. Sleep is impossible on this bumpy white-knuckle ride, dropping off the sides of each breaking wave with a shuddering slam in this near gale. The going is tedious so at 4am the decision is made to change our course and head for San Remo instead of Menton, that being nearer, safer and a better sailing angle.

At early dawn the lights of San Remo are vaguely discernable, the sea is quieter and we can begin to relax and enjoy a steadier sail. At 8.15am we gratefully come alongside the reception quay at Porto Sole marina in San Remo, and courteously assisted with the warps, not caring that it is expensive or that we've been here before.

After a distance of 103 nautical miles, never have the following bacon, eggs and coffee tasted so good! A siesta seems justifiable, before cycling to the supermarket to forage for supper. I think it is minced beef, but we are too tired to notice

The overall distance from La Ciotat is now 1,150.43 nm.

Chapter 6

Getting ourselves into gear this morning is a little slow, even so at 11.15am, having called at the fuel dock, we are out of the marina, with a light breeze wafting into the jib and mainsail as we flop along at three and a half knots, trying to dodge the fish pots in a rolling sea. Come lunch time, some smart Alec suggests heaving to.

Whether anyone actually eats their own lunch is doubtful, you just have to catch whatever slides past and as a result, 'chase the olives' becomes a new game.

Enough of rolling round, the jib is reset and a few tacks put in before motoring into the old harbour of Menton with hopes of being able to stay for a few days in the space we have found. As this has been only a gentle 14.2 mile passage with an average speed of 2.8 knots, we have not been exactly over-pressed, so are ready for some exploration.

Des, being a rugby fan tells us that William Webb Ellis, the founder of the game is buried in Menton, hence the afternoon is taken up with a pilgrimage to two cemeteries, both of which are up hundreds of uneven steps, through narrow streets and alley ways. After puffing our way up to the top of the town, we search through the ornate marble monuments displaying photographs of loved ones, tombs resembling sentry boxes, angels with broken wings and rusting wrought iron railings. We see graves of high ranking sea captains, many titled English gentle folk, World War 1 victims and Sir Walter Scott, but no William Webb Ellis.

In celebration of Sam's birthday we dine out modestly at La Merle Blanc, imbibing just the right amount of wine needed to test the hopscotch pitches that are marked out along the promenade gardens. Our antics raise a round of applause from a bemused threesome, whereupon one lady aims to upstage our display by hopping the full length of the pitch to end with a flourish by using the railings as a ballet barre. We think she may have had a sip of wine or two.

The birthday cards that Des brought with him for Sam are collected up again – we got the date wrong.

September 25th

Happy Birthday again Sam. The cards are re-issued then the rest of the morning is spent trying to organise Des's return home, renting a car and buying some meat for tonight's suggested barbecue. After Italy, it is a pleasure to see the great variety of pâtés, cheeses, meat and vegetables so beautifully displayed in the old, ornate food hall.

The lively, convivial atmosphere of the *Place Aux Herbes* invites us to sit in the shade of the plane trees, people-watching at the Lido bar and also being pestered to buy watches or trinkets from the oriental hawkers. A hire car is booked for tomorrow.

The boat barbecue has not yet been used so it needs a bit of attention and the damp charcoal has to be well fanned before it almost sets fire to the deck, but duly gives a good glow for the sausages and chicken. Mis-judging the amounts when making 'Hush Puppies' results in feeding the excess cornbread lumps to the children and their dog on the opposite boat. The wise dog breaks them up – is it for easier eating or to be able to push them between the gaps in the planking?

Keeping up our standards, the meal is graced with an impudent Rosé wine, delicately decanted from a one and a half litre plastic, screw top bottle, marked 12 francs.

September 26th

This day begins black and wet with the mountain tops shrouded in thick cloud, not ideal conditions for sightseeing but what can we do instead?

The hire car does not arrive and on phoning the office, we learn that it has been taken to the new port instead of the old one, where we are. When that is resolved, we are soon winging our way twice round the railway station, the square and several roundabouts before finding the way out of town.

The winding mountain roads up to the ancient, picturesque village of St Agnes has spectacular views of the coastline, breath taking scenery and gasp-making hair pin bends. The village is small with narrow streets and attractive toy town shops but it is now time for lunch. At the first restaurant we enter, a cat oblivious to customers is sitting on the tablecloth compulsively scratching each part of its anatomy in turn. The restaurant has the same type of cats but at floor level. It is staffed by a family of noticeably low aptitude, and the chef sets fire to our omelettes. (Is it the wine or inter breeding?)

The cloud, which had obscured the view on arrival has now cleared to reveal further panoramic scenery as we cling to our seats round more tight corners and into Peille. Here is a medieval communal wash house, fountain, memorial gardens and a charming central square backed by the *Marie*, or town hall.

Up even higher is Peillon, another tiny medieval village with two cosy hotels, a sculptor's studio and a fountain amongst a warren of narrow alleys. But no shops.

Heading back we pass La Turbie and the outskirts of Monaco to drive along the Grande Corniche and through Eze village, which is another little gem to be more fully explored some day.

Back in Menton with no inclination to start cooking, we pick up some hot quiche and fries that together with salad and a dab of local brew makes a fitting finish to a good day out, and a welcome change from a harbour wall.

September 27th

There is a Mistral blowing, the sky is very blue, it is cold and we are up early to make full use of the car before it has to be returned at 11.30am.

First we drive to Garavan marina to enquire about a winter mooring for *Kalivala* and the answer is a positive "Non!"

Des drops us off at St Michael's cemetery to save a long climb, returns the car and he is kindly brought back up to join us. This time the quest for the William Webb Ellis's grave is successful. The inscription reads:

William Webb Ellis
Who with a fine disregard for the rules of football
as played in his time
first took the ball in his arms and ran with it
Thus originating the distinctive feature of
the rugby game

In 1823 he became the Reverend of St Clement Danes.

Our mission accomplished, we take an easy walk down through the geranium-hung alleys into *Place Aux Herbes*, sitting outside in spite of the cold wind of the Mistral.

Today is different from usual, an antique fair is being held and the square is full of tables laden with trinkets and *objets d'art*. Suddenly, an extra strong gust rips through the archways and the scene becomes one of chaos and destruction. The tablecloths whip up, sending china plates crashing onto the concrete slabs, table lamps become air born along with books and wrapping paper A shout of "*Ferme la porte, s'il vous plait!*" (Close the door, please), can be heard above the tinkling of broken glass and pots as the stallholders hasten to rescue their wares. Between chuckles, we did have a smidgen of pity for the plight of madame who is caught whilst trying to pick up arms full of vases, when an extra strong playful gust blows her long dress right up over her head and she is quite unable to defend her *derrière!* The same voice is heard loudly requesting "*Montrez-moi votre pantalons encore!*" Which she helplessly obliged several times.

On our return, the ventometer is registering 41 knots of wind, a hasty re-adjustment to the warps and fenders is needed before lunch.

Our friend Des, packs up and is ready for the taxi he ordered for 5pm. At 5.20pm he panics and re-orders it. The taxi duly arrives at 5.35pm leaving us short of time for the station, when due to conflicting opinions between the Information Bureau and the guard, we are not sure if we put him on the right train. It has been fun having extra crew and it is sad to wave goodbye, wherever he is going.

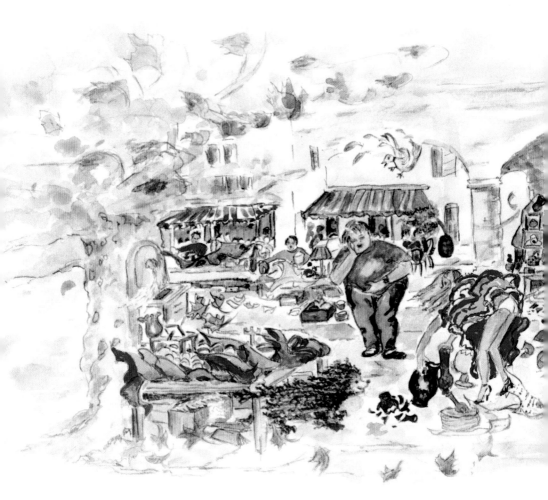

"Fermé la porte! Montrez-nous votre culottes encore."
Place aux Herbes in a Mistral

September 28th

Today begins sunny with a cool breeze. Catching the 10.42am train to Beaulieu, we go to the shipyard to make enquiries about the chances of a winter berth, and curtly learn that there is no chance at all, either in the water or out on the hard. We wait for a bus to St Jean Cap Ferrat, which fails to arrive so now the only way is to walk by the pleasant two mile coastal path which passes David Niven's elegant villa on a small wooded headland.

The shipyard here is courteous and helpful and a provisional booking is made to crane out *Kalivala* to store on the hard for six months - at a special price of course.

It now starts to rain, and lunch is taken under the awning of one of the many quayside restaurants where a surly waitress manages to foul up the orders. An American on the next table is served with Sam's ham omelette and chips, and before we could tell him he sends it back because he had ordered a cheese one, which after some delay, is heavily placed in front of him. With further delay Sam gets a ham and cheese one defiantly slapped down, and duly the chips arrive. It takes some time and concentration to think up the translation into French to convince *madame* that the order was for just a ham omelette and chips and that is what we wish to pay for.

By the time we walk back in the rain, catch the train and trudge back to the boat via the supermarket in a thunder storm, our legs are aching and it has seemed a very long day. The wind now blows straight into the harbour entrance, rolling all the boats like corks.

September 29th to October 15th
Partly due to the atrocious weather, but mainly because we enjoy Menton we stay on for a further sixteen days. Torrential rain, thunderstorms and strong winds alternate with short spells of perfect warm sunshine. Then we can swim beside the remaining German holiday makers loudly floundering in the shallows in their frilly bathing hats, along with the multi shaped, topless madamoiselles.

In contrast, the heavy rain causes chaos with the traffic and the shoppers. Caught in a squall, I aquaplane unexpectedly on the white stripe of a pedestrian crossing and land in a wet, undignified heap on the road with not a gallant Gall in sight to help pick up the rolling potatoes and apricots. The onlookers under their umbrellas enjoyed the diversion as I scrabble around to rescue my purchases, then gingerly return with my shoes in the other hand.

Meanwhile, the rain has seeped down some screw holes onto the bedding again and a Siamese cat has taken refuge from the storm in the saloon. The cat disappears down the back of the settee to somewhere inaccessible between the boarded lining and the fibre glass hull. "Oh dear. What a CATastrophy!"

However, the more pressing concern at present is with the wet bedding, so screws have to be tightened and sealed as quickly as possible. It is a fair time before we are relieved to notice a back leg and a kinked tail easing their way out from behind the seat, after a full boat inspection. The cat then makes itself at home as it curls up and sleeps on a cushion.

It has now rained non stop for 41 hours. In the harbour, a three-parts sunken motor boat is towed back in from having broken free from its moorings, and we are told by a local fisherman that others had sunk with the weight of water - and also that the clocks had been put back on winter time two days ago. We had not noticed any difference.

Each day has some domestic chores. Washing is usually done in buckets and bowls here, then it is festooned round the guard rails between showers. Replacing the small plugs in the teak decking is a never ending tedious task, and since Sam carves each one to fit only a few get done per week.

Shopping here is a pleasure, and the nice part is that the baguette always seems to need a rest as it comes to *La Place Aux Herbes*, and what better place is there than on a chair under the plane trees at Bar Lido? Here you can be entertained by puppets, pan pipes and pedlars, although the latter do not have much response trying to sell their beads, model cars and 'genuine' Rolex watches.

The next antique market suffered yet more rain. The vendors look very dejectedly at the bar clientele that sit stoically drinking their coffees, beers and kirs with the rain dripping down their necks from between the awnings. Sam observantly remarks, "At least it washes the doggo off the pavements."

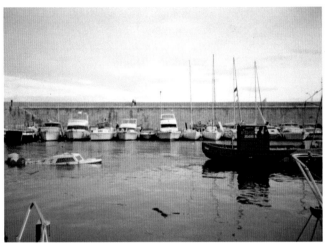

One of the casualties, Menton

The cat has been doing a daily kit inspection and making itself comfortable, but we cannot find out where it comes from.

On fine days the sea at 70° F is still warm enough for swimming but now, having adjusted to the hour difference, the sun dips down behind the mountain by 6pm leaving the sky colours graduating from deep blue to green, yellow and a deep rosy glow silhouetting the palm trees and little fortress behind us. As we sit with our own glow, we forget that the main intention was supposed to be for Greece, Turkey and beyond.

It is almost a pleasure to go to the bank here. The staff are suitably dressed and not in T-shirts, shorts and a dangling cigarette, no taking off belts and watches, and cheques are cashed instantly without having to join two queues. Left over lira are exchanged for French francs making us feel quite well off, until we post the deposit for the winter moorings.

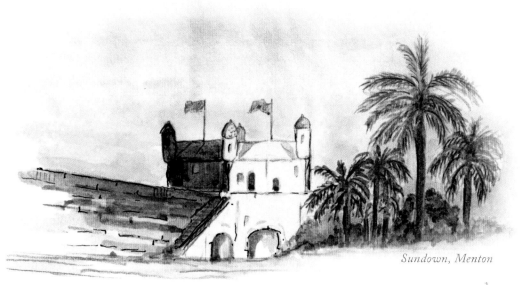

Sundown, Menton

The next intended call is the travel agent's, to find out about the best method to get home. Somehow we become side tracked into an estate agents instead, thinking that a place of our own seems an attractive idea. The first viewing is in the old town up endless uneven steps with no access for a car, then a flight of stairs reveals a nice view and suspicious plumbing for £68,000. The next is a spacious 7th floor flat for £70,000, this being disadvantaged by facing east, and is one and a half miles out of town. The third one is perfect, in an excellent sea view position but regrettably, has a few more noughts on the price. Due consideration is given to these properties whilst the baguette takes its rest at *The Lido*.

The baguette – resting!

"Why do we need a flat? There is adequate accommodation on the boat and we can move it if we become bored with the view." That settled, we take a spare GAZ bottle down to the supermarket where Madame Allari offers to sell it for us. Two days later she beamingly gives us 80 francs, which Sam promptly invests in his cellar, thus adding another Côtes de Roussillon and a Bordeau to his collection.

In the window of a Red Cross charity shop we notice a small electric heating element which could help to supplement the gas. It's extraction from the front of the window causes quite a disturbance amongst the jumble sale grabbing clients. It proves to be not one of our best ideas as it takes twenty minutes to boil two mugs of water, although turned on its side it gives out a highly dangerous, welcome bit of warmth. Tread carefully cat or you will go 'WOOF' instead of miaow.

One day there is a notice pinned to a tree advertising a free orchestral concert to be held in the *Palace de Europe* at 8.30pm as part of the 30th anniversary celebrations of Menton's twinning with the German town of Baden Baden.

Halfway through supper we think that it might be a good idea to go so hasten to make ourselves suitably presentable. The skirt is a bit crumpled with lack of use, trousers have a few extra creases and shoes are uncomfortable as we hasten to the lovely concert hall to find the last two rickety chairs upstairs on the jam shelf, just in time for the opening bars of the overture to *Carmen*. The orchestra is comprised of very young and very old players so although lacking in a little sparkle and polish, they still enthusiastically brave their way through an enjoyable programme. Bizet, Suppe and Strauss surrender to a funny little conductor resembling a clockwork beetle, who encourages several encores after clapping along with the *Annen Polka*.

More storms are howling in from the east straight into the harbour causing a swell, which pulls on the rusty, metal mooring springs making them groan and the warps sing like an orchestra tuning up. What a cacophony when the fenders join in with their squeaking. A cover is hastily fashioned from an old sweater for the large rowdy blue one, a smaller one bursts and flattens, and one is sawing through its cord so we tie on a few extra ones before abandoning the rocking horse motion for *terra firma*. Waves break over the wall, the fairy lights are being taken down on the promenade and there are no English newspapers; Menton is declaring 'End of season.' Should we be moving on or going home? The weather dictates that we must wait.

Sometimes it is possible to make phone calls on the VHF radio on board when we can check up on uncle's welfare and have family news, and we hear that Carl is wishing us to contact him at his office in La Ciotat. "Now what does he want?" In order to comply we have to wade through the deluge of yet another thunderstorm to the hotel St Michel, where a helpful receptionist allows the use of her desk telephone.

As suspected, "Would we like to help him sail his yacht *Olivia* (still in Bandol) back across the Atlantic?" That sounds interesting, it might be less hassle than trying to sail the next ten miles down this coast but it will not be until this time next year so, drink your coffee and don't worry about it now. Arrangements are made to visit him in Bandol for discussions.

On the few days that the sun shines for a while the town is busy, we can dry the washing and air bedding, but before long the menacing clouds build up over the mountains, the boats are restless again and the lightning highlights our efforts to quieten the noisy fenders.

The cat shows great displeasure by sinking its claws into my hand when being evicted but we need to ease the stern warps. The cat moans, spits and wags its tail as it tries to weigh up the possibility of a tight rope walk, then it gives up in disgust. Now we also have a longer jump. What happened to the plans of a new plank?

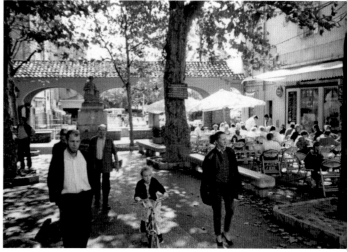

La Place aux Herbs. Bar Lido, Menton

October 14th Menton to St Jean Cap Ferrat

The rattle of beating rain, shrieking wind, thunder and all the accompanying orchestral sounds wake us early but in hopes of later improvement, we puddle jump down to the *Capitainerie*, pay our dues and donate a bottle of good wine as a small gesture of thanks. Sam gets the fidgets at lunchtime, and before I have eaten the last olive he has started the engine. It is NOT fit to leave, the horizon is ragged under heavy black cloud and the sea is not at all inviting, but the forecast for the next few days is even more forbidding, so we go!

As soon as we clear the harbour the pitching and tossing begins, there is not much wind and for once, it is not a head wind. No, it is straight up the stern. That, with a very disturbed quartering sea makes it a boring passage, alternating between surfing down waves and slewing round unexpectedly onto every point of the compass.

As it is only ten miles we had hoped that the last sail of the season would be a good one, but at least it is memorable especially as we are accompanied by two dolphins leaping and diving under the bows for most of the way.

Arriving at 3.15pm the *Capitaine* is more than a little surprised as we are not expected until the end of the month, but after a few minutes of shrugging and pondering, he manages to find us a harbour side berth with a grandstand view of all the happenings.

There is time to inspect the surroundings and find that St Jean is a small, pretty community on a wooded headland. There are adequate small shops, many restaurants along the quay and a general air of opulence – not the place to hang the washing on the guardrails.

Back on board there is a strange feeling. It is the silence and stillness, no screeching fenders or frapping halyards. Peace, that is until the church clock chimes midnight on its all four faces.

October 15th

Since *Kalivala* is not due to be lifted out of the water until the 28th it leaves plenty of leisure time, but first we must renew the *Constituto*, the permit required by the Customs Officials. In due course this is obtained at the third time of cycling through to Beaulieu.

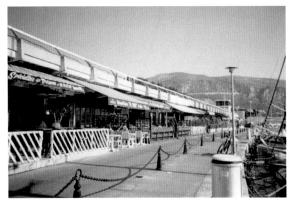

At the first call, the office is closed; the next time, the officer is heavily involved with a cruise ship, which due to the weather, has been forced to shelter in his bay instead of round the corner in Villefranche. Third time lucky, and we are legal again.

For the visit to Bandol, the trains prove to be too complicated so we hire a car and enjoy a scenic drive through the mountains, arriving in the late afternoon. To our surprise there are several of the La Ciotat office staff on Carl's boat and not the prospective crew for an Atlantic crossing. Why? It seems that this gathering is to enable Carl to introduce everyone to Bella. Wife number five.

Everybody is taken out to dine before we spend a very cold night on board his renamed boat, *Hope*.

First thing Carl cooks up a mound of breakfast, then whisks us off to Cassis to show Bella the villa where I had idled whilst waiting for Sam. Apart from an iron and ironing board, it looked as bare as ever. From there he takes us to Aix en Provence, an interesting town but the only purpose seems to be for them to buy a book and a length of highly expensive material, although we do have a brief glimpse of the fountains and Roman Forum in passing. It is very cold even when sitting under an electric heater outside in the restaurant awning for lunch.

Back in Bandol, we have to amuse ourselves walking round town in the freezing wind as the two love birds said they needed a rest. Oh, the bliss! Sitting next to the pizza oven in a little Italian bistro where Mama declares her love for Sam.

Back on board *Hope* we sneak about until we find two extra blankets and sleep soundly. The word Atlantic has not once been mentioned. Why are we here?

October 16th

The drive back to St Jean Cap Ferrat is rather slow due to frequent stops at the spectacular viewpoints, appreciating the very blue sea against red rocks, snow topped mountains and the pine and eucalyptus trees. The traffic through Nice and Cannes causes more delay, leaving no time to visit Vence as hoped.

The hired car has to be returned to Beaulieu, there we unsuccessfully try to find out about train and ferry times, before walking back along the ever enjoyable coastal path.

Some other paths we have discovered are even nicer. Towards the headland in the opposite direction, there are imposing residences. One such is the Villa

Mora, a pink confection resembling an iced birthday cake, then a modest castle tucked away behind walls of trailing bougainvillea. A little further on is a small pebble beach backed by an inviting restaurant, and beyond that, pine woods opening up onto a rocky promontory where, one day a very English voice calls out "Bit like Cornwall – innit?"

The other side of the peninsula is not quite so pleasant. What had been little summer houses with barbecues, are now derelict and unsightly and the rocks are like a moonscape leading onto a long concrete path. This we surmise is the cover up for the sewage system flowing directly in to the sea, hence this route becomes termed as the Effluent Way, and is avoided.

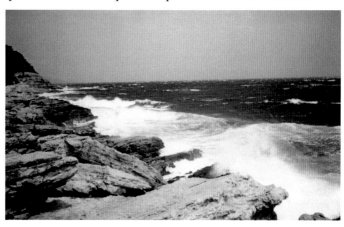

The sea throws up a few useful finds - a good washing up bowl, a fishing line with a float and two hooks, and a small fender. It is quite disturbing to notice the trivial things that we get excited about now; I think we are missing the anticipation of arriving at each different port, the frights, tensions and humorous incidents. This life seems quite tame, but on the other hand we don't have screwed up stomachs and are regaining the weight we have lost.

The evenings are full of the buzz, chatterings and clatterings of the adjacent bars and restaurants, lasting well into the night as the accordionists serenade every table at each establishment.

October 24th

Since arriving in St Jean, we have been befriended by many people, both English and French, perhaps because we are on the front row so many stop to chat.

There is the couple touring in a very small camper van to whom we lent our key to the shower block, they return the favour by bringing over their bottle of Drambui and four glasses. An ex-naval commander and his wife kindly offer a flow of unnecessary advice and Bob, three boats away offers to take us and our luggage to the station when we are ready to go home. We enjoy this sociable position on the quayside for the next few days.

At last the train is booked for us to return home on October 31st, but the travel agent cannot oblige with ferry tickets so we return to the station. The clerk almost dives under the counter when he sees us again and keeps his telephone call going as long as possible before deigning to acknowledge us, being a bit at a loss dealing with *Les Anglais*. After a long process on the computer, he makes a reservation on the Calais to Dover ferry which satisfactorily connects with the trains, and we all heave a sigh of relief. Then follows a flurry of activity between intermittent storms, lovely sunny days and pine wood walks, as we set about making preparations for returning home.

Do we really need all these tatty T-shirts and underwear? One full bag is loaded into the back of Bob's rusting, dinted old estate car and it sags a little – wait till we get the rest. The whole boat is scoured before finding the purse containing the reserve of English money, resulting in a few cupboards being cleaned and tidied – what do we do with all this pasta that is left over from the Italian influence when there was nothing else we had confidence in? Put it back in the cupboard and go for a walk whilst the sun is shining – the white foam against the turquoise and aquamarine of the curling waves are much more appreciated when you are not out there battling against its turbulence.

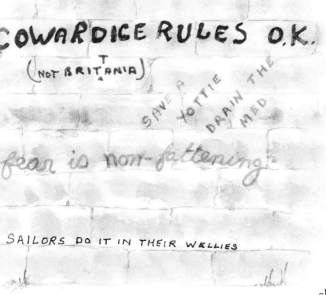

A wall in St John Cap Ferrat - very out of keeping

October 27th

More rain and a big sea out of all proportion to the light wind inspires more cupboard cleaning, whilst Sam removes the Wallis heater and ailing fridge motor to put into Bob's car for repair at home, together with the rented life raft and a box of bits. (Dare we mention the other spare gas bottle?) The car's back end sags even more.

Feeling that Carl should be reminded that we shall be at home for the winter, we ring his La Ciotat office, only to learn that he has gone back to his Florida premises. The pain of the expensive few minutes phone call from the booth in the Voile d'Or hotel is lightened by the display of autographed photographs of Roger Moore, Rex Harrison, Jack Nicholson, J.R. Ewing and numerous other well known film stars. Perhaps they are the friends of David Niven who lives just along the promenade. And here we are in our work clothes.

October 28th

Today *Kalivala* is being lifted out onto the hard standing area. Fortunately the heavy seas have abated making it easy to motor straight into the lifting bay under the travelling crane, where it is efficiently lifted promptly at 10am to be placed in position on blocks and props, and given a high pressure hose down. It is surprising to see how little growth of algae there is on the hull after a year in the water. There are just a few patches of worm-like Crustacea, which easily scrubs off.

Another surprise later, and a disconcerting one is that our ensign has been spat on. It is unusual that in this good class, apparently friendly area, there is some resentment of boat owners or dislike of the British being felt by unknown persons.

It is a strange feeling to be high up, perfectly motionless and with no squeaking fenders, but it's just a pest that the security spotlight points directly down the aft cabin hatch all night, reminding us of battery hens.

October 29th

A busy morning, floor boards are taken up to mop out the bilges revealing dust, fluff, crumbs and oily gunge. Then Sam starts to polish the hull watched by a husky type dog with shifty pale blue eyes. Its owners, also working on their boat are a very friendly pair of Cockneys with a very coarse, humorous turn of phrase which helps to lighten the chores with their interruptions.

Most marinas have the sneaky practice of removing the sink plugs and making the hot taps inoperable. A week's laundry is accomplished by filling up the newly found washing up bowl with scalding water from the showers and using the cap off the washing up liquid as a plug. I must not complain too much about these facilities as the toilets do have seats and tissue as you would expect, but very few facilities do.

Now there is some fibre-glass filling and plastic padding repairs to make a mess with round the keel and skeg, being the results of a few miscalculations of depth and the occasional sunken, abandoned shopping trolley. The dinghy, oars, outboard engine, life belts, the two bicycles and other sundry deck ornaments are stowed and everywhere begins to look tidy and ship shape.

This is all very thirsty work and we are down to the last bottle of beer, one carrot, half an onion and a noggin of high powered cheese, but there is no point in buying more now.

October 31st St Jean Cap Ferrat to home in Hamble

Excitement is tinged with a little sadness as Bob takes us to the station, his aging motor groaning under the weight of two more bodies, four holdalls plus the objects previously stowed.

Somehow, we manage to hump the life raft, fridge motor, heater and the four heavy bags on and off three trains and the ferry to be thankfully met by car for the last leg of the journey to Hamble.

How long will it be before the novelty of television, hot baths and plentiful water wears off?

Chapter 7

Small portion of Irish Stew

May 12th Return to St Jean Cap Ferrat

It is time again to leave the cosy pastime of homes and gardens and head back to life at sea and wisely or foolishly, take the car to transport the overhauled heater, fridge motor, Marmite, salad cream, too many clothes and a pile of books.

The cross channel passage on the *Duc de Normandy* is a rough one, slowing down progress and passengers are not allowed on deck. By the time the port entrance is reached in Ouistreham, the tide has ebbed too far and the ferry runs aground to the sound of churning engines and jeering passengers – and we think our navigation is a bit slapdash. It is almost an hour before it reaches port and we can begin to motor down France, passing through Le Mans, Tours, Clermont Ferrant and making over night stops at Mayet and Florac, all in pleasantly rural countryside.

Kalivala has wintered well; it is dry inside but feels a bit strange to be back. During the next few days, the sails are hanked back on, the refrigerator motor installed, the bikes pulled out of the aft cabin and between bouts of deck scrubbing and two thunderstorms, we reacquaint ourselves with the shops and *Le Yacht* bar.

May 19th

In two days time a couple of close friends will be arriving for a holiday on board with us, but right now the wind is howling and the sea is pounding over the sea wall, making all the boats wallow. Oh dear! They will wish they had gone to Scotland instead!"

After a very domesticated morning, we decide to check the car in case sailing is not an option. Something is wrong here – the doors are unlocked and the radio has been wrenched and broken in an attempt to remove it. There had been a few furtive-looking lads loitering around last night.

Our walk now is to the Gendarmerie where we try to explain the incident to an acne'd underling warily twitching his gun in his holster, whilst three other junior gendarmes wrestle with a very irate handcuffed, Irishman. They are not quite sure what to do with him as he rant, flails, kicks and swears in his colourful patois. Then we become caught up in the verbal crossfire as he rounds his wrath onto us. *Mad Mick* is loudly insisting that we are British and should be witnesses to this treatment. Between oaths, outbursts and struggles, he tries to wheedle us to roll him a cigarette, but a more senior gendarme behind him is wagging a finger and shaking his head to tell us not to do so.

He continues to rant to us about "...working on deck, picking up me knife and putting it in me pocket ... and I swear on me grandmother's grave, they dragged me off the f***ing bus and handcuffed me. I'll find you. I will. I'll look till I find you, and make you f***ing witnesses, begorrah!"

This is all rather disconcerting, since we are only here to report a break-in, which alone is sufficiently worrisome.

We look anxiously from Mick to the gendarmes, not sure whether they understand what he is implying then somehow, they manage to forcibly persuade him into another office and we are able to deal with the matter in hand. This needs a return to the boat for passports, ship's papers, claim forms and almost size of shoes, before a letter can be typed to our Insurance Company. It is then that a much chastened, even smiling Mick appears without hand cuffs and bids us a cheery goodbye.

Two other men, who have apparently resolved his problem accompany him, and one explains to us that, "Just a belligerent Irishman celebrating his mother's birthday!"

Anyway, I suppose it made an interesting afternoon considering we were only going as far as the Hotel Voile d'Or to watch the waves breaking over the sea wall into their swimming pool.

May 22nd
Yesterday, before meeting our friends, Noel and Anne off the train, we priced the gang planks in consideration for them. £400! Sorry, you will just have to jump as we do. They say they are agog for an action packed, exciting holiday, and it to start immediately.

Fortunately, they are both experienced sailors but this gives rise to some barracking in the cockpit as we roll along like a drunken pig in a disturbed swell for ten miles to back track once more into Menton.

Now that we know the way, we lead them up the endless steps to impress them with the grave of William Webb Ellis of rugby fame, ignoring Noel's complaints about the lack of oxygen at such an altitude.

Back down at sea level, it is necessary to rest in the familiar *Place aux Herbes* to treat his imaginary dehydration brought on by the ascent.

May 23rd Menton to Villefranche
On a calm sea, this fourteen mile sail is most enjoyable, and even the two skippers are not arguing about the course. On the way we slowly waft in and out of Monte Carlo where all the big boy's expensive toys bob gently on the pontoons and the road barriers and stands are being erected in readiness for the famous road races.

Arriving in Villefranche, Sam surprises us all by making a perfect reverse into a narrow slot on the harbour wall just as the sun comes over the yardarm. The luxury motor cruiser *Ghislaine*, once belonging to the ill fated Robert Maxwell is moored nearby awaiting its destiny.

In the attempt to keep our guests occupied all day, we show them the Rue Obscura - 'a dark tunnel under the houses' is Noel's description of it. Next we take them to see the Volti sculptures in the old ramparts, which he considers rather rude, and his lip still quivers when he sees the sketch. From there we puff up several flights of steps to the park to criticise yet more similar sculptures and carry on to the castle museum. This houses a totally forgettable exhibition of modern art, which is briefly huffed at before coming across a spirited boules match, giving a welcome excuse to sit down and watch. Distances of one finger or half a finger between the boules are bickered over with great humour, dramatic gestures and much heckling. On the way back, our two menfolk are intrigued by some music drifting through a door on which a notice says *La salle notre dame de toutes les joies*, and consider its merits as a possible evening venue to find out just what 'all the joys' are. As it happens, apathy rules and instead we are passably entertained by a nearby industrious man with an electric drill over-riding the restaurant tenor as he fights his tormented way through *Tosca*.

May 24th

The next six days are spent sailing up and down the coast, mostly to places already known to us and staying overnight in marinas at Cannes, St Tropez, Port Grimaud, St Maxime, Antibes, Napoule then back to St Jean. The weather is a tolerable mixture of sun, cloud, lumpy sea or flat calm, with each day only involving only two or three hours at sea and a fair time of that spent listening to the two men disputing the course to steer – not that it really mattered, the coastline was never far away; we only covered 132.76 nautical miles all week!

Noel meets Volti

Each night, the virtues of a few local wines are discussed in depth to blot out the night noises of the tinkling piano bar in conflict with the Oom-pah band who are competing with the accordions next door and not forgetting the jangling halyards and the planes landing at Nice airport.

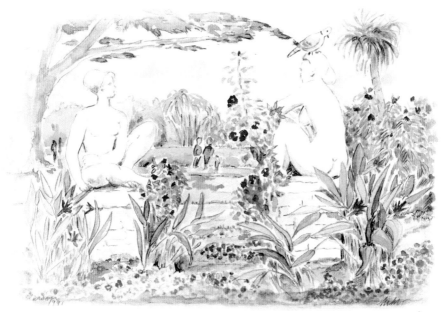

Keep your eyes shut, Cherie

May 30th

Heavy low cloud dispels all thoughts of sailing, so we take advantage of the car and drive along the *Moyenne Corniche* up to the charming village of Eze where Noel is shamed into climbing yet more steps up to the unusual cactus garden. The views across the bay to St Jean make all the effort worthwhile. Just outside the village are the two perfumeries, Galinard and Fragonard so how could we resist the free tour and all the sampling? Together with the spectacular scenery and four bodies each exuding a mixture of several potent perfumes, the journey back is a very heady experience. This lasts well into the night until lulled by the hum of voices from the restaurants and their clatterings and - *boy, do we smell good!*

May 31st

No sailing again today instead, another white knuckle ride up countless hairpin bends and a *route dangereuse* to the small ancient communities of La Turbie and Peille. Vibrant purple bougainvillea clashes with the orange nasturtiums that hang down over the narrow cobbled streets leading to the Roman columns on the Triumphe de Augustus, archways, fountains and a notable amount of doggo.

The visit is brief as we have to take our friends into Nice to catch their train home. The traffic is hectic, we are late and there is nowhere to park, and the only thing we can do is just bundle them out at the station and shout, "Goodbye," whilst the cars hoot impatiently behind us – not the way we wished their holiday to end.

Monaco radio announces that the Monte Carlo Grand Prix has been won by Ayrton Senna and just lost by Nigel Mansell because of an unlucky tyre change shortly before the end of the race.

It is strangely quiet tonight

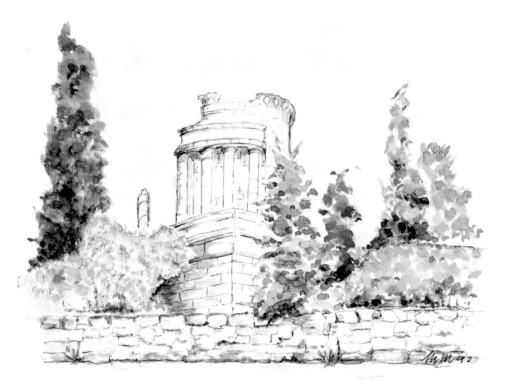

Triumphe d'Augustus, La Turbie

June 1st
There is no barracking and plenty of room round the breakfast table this morning, but we do miss them. Intentions of going to the launderette are thwarted by the Australian lady opposite, who calls across requesting any spare reading matter. After she talks incessantly for half an hour, I off load two thick, tatty, rather boring paperbacks and a week old newspaper. Since she had nothing to give in return, I think she fared quite well. By this time the clouds have gathered bringing rain and thunder, and the laundry is postponed.

June 2nd
As there is not the enthusiastic urge to reach the next destination now, we can blend in with the community and enjoy the local events for as long as the *Capitaine* will permit.

The family would like another holiday with us in July, and as this is a good place to meet them, we wheedle another month's stay here; the cravings for Greece and Turkey are long gone. Domestic issues such as the ongoing hammering of teak deck plugs, and decorating the guardrails with washing have to be dealt with.

Sam de-crusts the lime scale from the thermostat on the engine, which might have accounted for the occasional overheating, then we drive into Nice to find a car radio shop. Prices are required so that we complete and send off the insurance claim. The search for a suitably priced boarding plank continues.

On one of our daily walks, we see a discarded refrigerator outside the gates of the little castle. Without conscience or regret, we did not resist the temptation to strip it of the rubber seal round the door in hopes of improving the efficiency of our own half hearted appliance, which is like a deep cool box where all the contents fall into a heap. To hopefully further its improvement, Sam buys a plastic foam spray for added insulation, which causes a snow storm in the under sink cupboard – thank goodness for lunchtime.

An oil change is the next messy task. When the right shop is duly found, we come out £20 lighter in purse into a sudden downpour, to dash across to a filter shop. Madame apologises for not being able to find the size we need and also for her highly smelly dog, which growls threateningly by her feet and, judging by its contortions, the dog is also home to fleas.

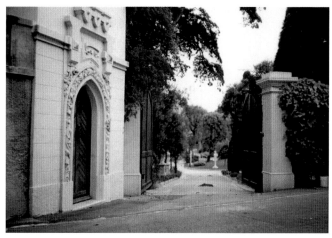

Gates of the little castle

After being sent twice more with queries to the smelly dog shop, madame eventually finds the correct filter. I then have the pleasure of tipping five wine bottles of old oil into a huge tank, which splashes it back into my face. Then I am required to donate the hard cover of my sketch book in order to make a new gasket.

There frequently seems to be some kind of event taking place here, helping us to integrate into the local life. The little art gallery has some garish weird paintings. I am intrigued to know what stories are behind them so I stop to talk to the little old lady artist. She is very charming, and having spent some of her childhood in Devon, tells me in perfect English that there are no stories, no preconceived ideas and no initial pencil drawings. "I just paint whatever comes to mind, so it is a surprise to me too." Well, you can see that, they are a surprise to anyone but she is delighted to have someone take an interest in her work. Personally, I would not put one of her pictures in an outside privy.

Saturday is market day in Beaulieu and we cycle in to soak up the colourful atmosphere. A slight calamity occurs when loading up the basket on my handlebars and the plastic box on the pannier. The overloaded bike suddenly loses its centre of gravity, turns and falls over whilst still chained up. Eggs collide with beer bottles, and the apples and potatoes take a slow roll across the tarmac as I am frustratedly trying to unlock the tight, twisted safety chain to release it from the 'No Parking' pole. Luckily, only one potato becomes pulp under a car wheel and everything else is retrieved undamaged.

One coastal path we follow, leads to a warm sheltered beach. *Plage Passable*, where a few brave souls are swimming and sunning themselves. Sam deems it passable as he views the bronzed bodies splayed on the sand.

Back on our side of the peninsula it is much cooler, and the dark clouds gather as we sit in the cockpit watching the waves slam over the sea wall and the strollers watching us. Then comes the rain again and 'Omar Shariff', the waiter at *Le Yacht* bar, is looking very miserable at the thought of fewer tips tonight as the menu boards blow over with a loud crash and the rain drips through the awning onto the tablecloths. Even the jolly Germans on the adjacent boat have stopped laughing because some of their crew are ill and they want to go home.

St Jean
Cap
Ferrat

There comes a few warmer days to enjoy. It is nicer than mowing lawns and housework, and even the fridge is responding slowly with an added ventilator in a cupboard door. The floor is taken up to insert a length of new piping for a hot water system, and as it all looks too technical I am glad of an excuse to escape, even if it is to visit the dentist again. An extra crusty piece of baguette has taken its toll on an old filling and an appointment has been made.

The session is not quite as expected for this supposedly upmarket area. There is no receptionist or dental nurse and I am handed the sucker to hold for myself. The dentist, a young Vietnamese lad dons a mask, visor and a pair of large yellow Marigold gloves before getting his head almost into my mouth. For the next twenty minutes I listen to the drill and try not to drown myself when distracted by his three year old son playing on the floor. He smiles as he requests 300 francs – "But it is porcelain, Madame."

The beach is now more often frequented and Sam is lured down one hot afternoon for a first swim. Men are not always very stoic. He complains that at 67^0 the water is too cold, and that he can't sit comfortably when trying to read with one eye and trying to conduct a thoracic survey with the other. Then he feigns a nonchalant, "When you've seen one, you've seen them all."

One breakfast time it is decided that this will be an alcohol free day, which results in spending more on substitutes and drinking apple juice at lunchtime. Strange ideas come into your head when it is clear of alcoholic pollution so, "How about an afternoon sail, just to show that we are not cemented to the wall?"

Apart from some power boats churning up the water, it is a tranquil short passage up as far as Eze sur Mer where a few tacks are made before freeing off and drifting gently back. I manage to make a good reverse entry into our berth – albeit at the second attempt.

The yacht full of jolly Germans who we thought had gone, come laughing back with a goodly bump into the wall, then spend the evening cleaning, shouting, polishing, laughing and scrubbing, before they donate some butter and cream to us and leave for a twelve hour drive back to Munich.

June 16th

From a phone call to the family, we learn that Carl wants Sam to ring him at the La Ciotat office again. What can he want this time? Although Sam is retired, he is still acting as a consultant when necessary so suddenly, on command we are preparing to drive the 130 miles over there. Nicely timed. We arrive for lunch then Sam spends several hours at the office whilst I am left with Carl's latest wife Bella, and as she does not want to miss her exercise class I am unsuitably kitted out in oversized white silky tights under a black swimsuit and dare not look in the mirror.

The hour of cruel stretch contortions is most painful - so it must be doing me some good. After a tasty supper at Carl's favourite Italian restaurant, we sleep in Bandol on his lovely yacht with the dodgy plumbing. Then as suddenly as we had left St Jean, we are on our way back again next morning, thinking "What a waste of time that was."

Returning by a prettier and more rural route, we dally at a vineyard to have a lesson on wine tasting in perfect English. Madame happily sells us several litres but the Winchester bottle container needed, costs almost as much as her 15 franc per litre wine.

"Oh, look. There's a wood yard." In the middle of nowhere is the long-sought-after plank. It costs less than £5, but with just the slight problem that it will not fit into the car boot. This is solved by opening the sun roof and resting it between us, then it protrudes a metre out of the top. This is almost satisfactory until we reach the mountains when, on every hairpin bend it slides from side to side batting us alternately across the ears and has to be uncomfortably held in place. I can now feel the results of yesterday's exercises. A *Bricomart*, the French equivalent of our B&Q comes in sight, where a number of accessories for the plank are found, so it doesn't seem such a waste of time after all.

June 20ᵗʰ

Many events are to take place during next week to celebrate the festival of the patron saint of St John. This starts with a charity run, which just happens to finish below the balcony of a very nice flat we have been invited to for the evening. The view is splendid, but we are driven inside by the tinny tannoy, cheering and loud music.

Much later the nearby pizzeria is in party mode, regaling its eaters with a guitarist who chokes on some Neapolitan love songs and is helped out with the choruses amid much applause. As a *grande finale*, an illuminated helicopter loudly chops past dangling a firework display on an unreadable plaque – could it be the St Jean coat of arms?

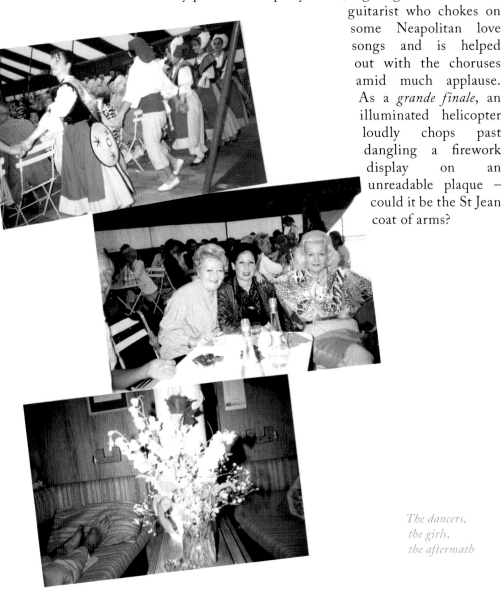

*The dancers,
the girls,
the aftermath*

June 21ˢᵗ Sunday

The town is celebrating again, starting with Mass in the huge marquee on the car park followed by a service at a monument to honour those who died in WW1 and WW11.

On the promenade, a *Magnifique* classic car exhibition is advertised. This consists of two Panhards, one MGA, a 1930 Packard, one Citroen, one Mercedes Benz, one Fiat and a Lassiter. They are all beautifully restored and gleaming. Then it starts to rain so we cross over to the marquee. The dancing is due to begin there at 11.45am, and since we are only dressed in shorts, we can shelter from the rain. We hesitate – there are attendants at the entrance. Do we need tickets? No, they beckon us in and we are surprised to see, not rows of seats as expected but chairs grouped round tables set with serviettes and plastic cups. Three other long tables have linen tablecloths and vases of flowers. People wearing smart suits and badges wander in to take their places at the long tables. "Oh, dear. What are we gate crashing now?" A few enquiries assure us that we are very welcome to this free municipal bash, courtesy of the Mayor.

Since we have nothing better in mind for a wet lunchtime, we hide our bare legs under a table for six, watching and waiting. Three people join us, the first introduces himself as a radio commentator and is with his wife, the other is a Colonel who insists on showing us his photograph album of aerial shots taken from his private aeroplane We try to look politely impressed, and keep quiet about ourselves. The colourful regional dancing begins, and just as we are feeling a bit out of depth, our three table guests depart and are promptly replaced by three predatory local sirens.

Dutifully we listen to the Mayor's speech, applauding when everyone else does. He welcomes the Mayors' of Villefranche, Beaulieu and Cap d'Ail, (the only remaining communist Mayor, and is not wearing a tie). Also welcomed are the guests of honour, who are the officers and crew from a naval minesweeper that is just back from the Gulf War. Bouquets are presented, more applause, then trays of food start to appear. Our table is served with two large plates of pizza slices, quiche squares and a bottle of wine. The friendly 'floosies' are perturbed – the other tables have two bottles. The dark eyed Algerian girl puts a hand out to a passing waiter and hijacks another bottle, and we all get talking. Three plates of chick pea pancakes and more quiche are set down, the blonde at our table waylays another bottle and we all start laughing. Sam now gets the hang of the game and extracts two more bottles from the tray of a distracted waiter, and we all become very happy – or words to that effect.

By this time the marquee is almost empty, and the cleaners are at work - perhaps it is time to go. Huegette, the other blonde clears the tables of flowers and shares them out as we leave at 4pm.

Out into the rain, the fairground is thronging with young hopefuls trying to win teddy bears from the crafty grabber crane and later, the Jazz and Rock Festival tries to burst a few eardrums. Thankfully we are far enough away not to grumble; we have had our excitement for today.

June 22nd

Sam pronounces this another alcohol free day. I wonder why?

A carpenter who will plane our plank for us has been located in a little narrow back street. We create a bit of a nuisance carrying it between us along several streets to his workshop, where he regards it through his bottle bottomed spectacles, and mutters, *Demain. Dix heures.* (Tomorrow. Ten o'clock.)

In the square, the big marquee has been packed up and the fairground stalls are battened down, all except for the one with the crane, which is still trying to catch a few more francs by dropping the teddy bears.

At mid day on *Radio Riviera*, we are surprised to hear a broadcast by Dieta Fredericks, the man we met yesterday. His subject – Travel tips.

An afternoon swim is a bit too refreshing and needs a walk afterwards to restore the circulation. The path marked *Privé* leads up past the lovely back gardens of affluent villas hidden among the trees, then down onto the rocks and back along the now deserted beach.

There is never a shortage of evening entertainment as we relax in the cockpit, and tonight our ears are assailed by a different accordionist serenading the diners at *Le Skipper* nearby. Judging by the half hearted applause, his attempts at *Zorba's Dance* and *By yon bonnie banks*, with half the notes missing does not impress them greatly.

June 24th

We awake to the sounds of heavy rain, a cracking thunderstorm and an evil smell near the refrigerator. The latter proves to be caused by an overlooked broken egg swimming in a leakage of beer and some stale bread, which was meant for the collared doves. What a bedraggled looking lot they are with their wet feathers. Some are limping and being bullied by a large fat dry one who had found a sheltered branch and is defending it.

This evening is the grand closing celebration of the St Jean Festival week. Supper is a little earlier tonight to be ready for the finale of this important local event. There is a 'crowd' of at least fifteen people gathering near the church, so it is obvious that something exciting is imminent. At 9pm a bell begins to toll, then a procession descends the church steps and here come six young choirboys about nine or ten years old, wearing short, shapeless surpluses of varying shades of whiteness, and trainers.

The first one is carrying a cross, not proudly but rather as if he is a bit embarrassed about it all and tries to pretend it is not there. The others just chatter, not really looking where they are going as they jostle and trip over their shoelaces. The priest solemnly follows then behind him come a few of the next stages of boyhood pushing a contraption on wheels. This is decorated with artificial leaves and carries a boom box, and a crackling loudspeaker belts out a *Trumpet Voluntary*.

Assorted members of the village congregation shuffle along behind to complete the grand procession, which is presided over by the Mayor. It is difficult not to

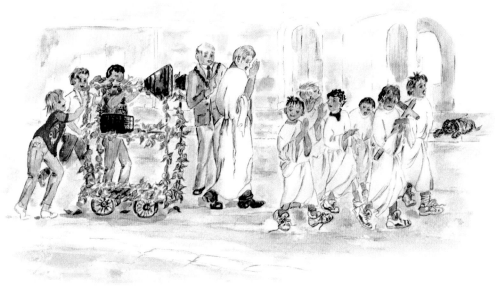

The Festival of St Jean

smile just a little and seem discourteous, especially when we turn to answer an English couple standing next to us who ask, "What was that?"

In conversation we ask them back to the boat for coffee, and have a grandstand view of the firework display that consists of five rockets and a ship's flare accompanied by a few hooters. St Jean certainly knows how to celebrate! All the same, it is charmingly unsophisticated and enjoyable. Several more social hours are spent with the two Brits during the next week of their holiday.

Between times, Sam is adorning the boarding plank with non slip strips, wheels and ropes for a handrail – it might have been as cheap to have bought a ready made *passerelle*.

On fair days we go out for a sail, but the popular anchorage is becoming so crowded with power boats and their toys, making it tricky to find space to drop anchor, and it is often less hassle to just heave-to half a mile off shore. There, we tie a fender on the end of a line to grab when swimming or take it in turns to be pleasantly towed along.

A wedding party has their reception in *Le Yacht*. The music sounds good at 7pm, even better at 8pm then at 11pm come the waltzes played on the typical French accordion - all very jolly. By 12.30 am it is a little tiresome, and at 3.45am we just wish they would all go home.

June 29th

Today we congratulate ourselves on the forty second anniversary of our marriage and wonder what we can do that is a bit different, but first we must go to the bank.

During a long queue there, I get talking to a tearful English lady. It seems that the flat she booked from an upmarket lady's magazine, is too unacceptably scruffy and dirty. She needs to be relocated but must pay in full again - it makes us very thankful to have the boat.

Due to the one way system, and in spite of a good map we still succeed in driving twice round Nice before finding the road to Levens, as suggested by the girl in the tourist office. On the way we stop for a potent coffee at a rather uninspiring café in which the only noteworthy feature is the toilet, which is on a balcony overhanging a river, making us wonder if they have bothered with the intricacies of plumbing when in the river is probably where every thing goes anyway.

The town of Levens is not overwhelming but it seems to make grand issue of all its previous Mayors and celebrities. There are plaques everywhere honouring flautists, tambourine players, artists, war heroes, Cistercian monks, lawyers and politicians. In the central square, we lunch on omelettes and beer whilst musing about, "What is black and brown, has four legs and flies?" The café Alsatian, and "what is white, has four wobbly legs and flies?" The café table.

Having looked at the gloomy chapel of the Black Penitento, noted for its paintings of the Fourteen Stations of the Cross we are drawn to a sign to *Maison du Portals* advertising an art exhibition. Up steps and narrow ally ways is the old house – this looks more interesting, but it is closed. As we turn to go away a breathless lady calls out, "Don't go away. I am just opening it up." We have no option now but to view it.

What an unexpected gem of an exhibition it is! Downstairs are small bronze action figures depicting family life by the Dutch artist, Kees Verkade. Upstairs are what were first thought to be just pleasing, modernistic figures, however, a closer look shows that they are all cleverly made from old farm implements. A group of hammer heads are so arranged to resemble a mother, or teacher, reading to children. Half a cow bell makes a flowing skirt for an elegant lady, old dessert spoons become herons and two crane hooks are so entwined to depict embracing lovers. Axe heads and sickles are imaginatively transformed by the artist, Jean Pierre Hugier, then bronzed and textured, making you want to touch them. Interspersed, are superb flower arrangements, intricate embroideries and fine quilting – even Sam is impressed.

An hour soon passes and as we leave, on turning to wave to the lady I step into something that needs washing off in the fountain. Why don't they have more control over their dogs, it is not easy to admire the scenery while having to watch where you are walking.

Driving back down the mountain roads, at an elevation of two thousand feet, we stop to listen to the silence and admire the profusion of wild flowers in the lush meadows. There are sweet peas, Canterbury bells, clovers, poppies, scabious and many other unrecognised species in such a riot of colour that puts our back garden to shame.

Back to reality, dodging through the frenzied traffic of Nice and then back to our cockpit where the setting sun glints tranquilly through the bottom of a glass. "Not a bad day out, was it ? At least we will remember it."

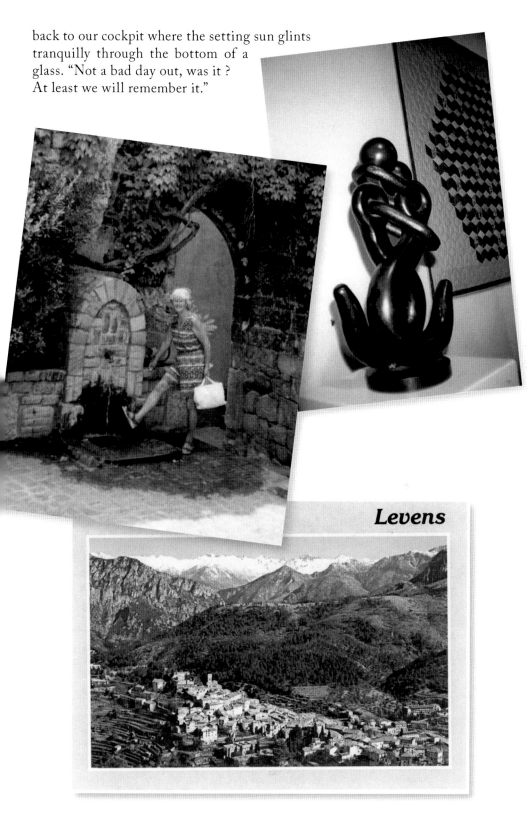

Levens

July 1ˢᵗ

The first highlight of today is to find a length of almost new, white nylon rope beside the dustbin, it had become a little grubby and must have been thrown away. Leaving the rope to soak, we cycle into Beaulieu for the market, pausing on return to pass comment on the newly erected, weird and whimsical sculptures in the park.

Waiters are prowling, looking for custom but halt to watch us as we scrub the length of rope, all sixty useful feet of it stretched out along the quay.

In the late afternoon, having walked in the rain to avoid having to sit below we become aware of some activity outside the *Salles des Fêtes*, just along the quay. Tables are put out with the familiar plastic cups and serviettes, then restrained applause is heard. This needs investigating. "Come on Sam, tuck your shirt in. I think it is another of the Mayor's binges."

To be precise it is the grand opening of the Art and Sculpture Exhibition, under the high patronage of Monsieur Vesti, Mayor of St Jean, Counsellor General of Alpe Maritime, all of which sounds most impressive. We go along to mingle and are rewarded with several plastic cupfuls of Vin Petillant and more slabs of quiche as, together with a few others we view the small collection of crude nudes, landscapes, blue horses, the Wailing Wall and suntanned backsides. The other critics are more interesting. There is the sad looking lady in a wet plastic anorak with matching miserable dog, a voluptuous has-been glamour girl garbed in black and white spotted everything, with gold boots

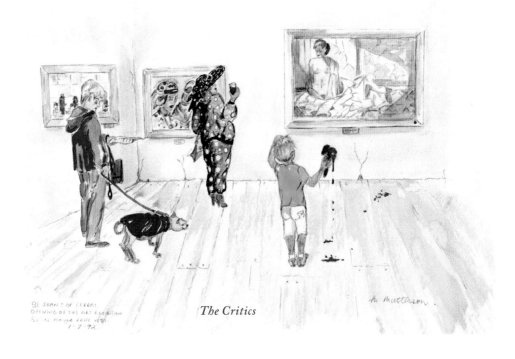

The Critics

and matching handbag. She slurps four cups of wine whilst gazing at one painting. Then there is a little boy, who drips his double strawberry ice cream as he tries not to look too interested in the life sized draped nude, revealing more than necessary in her uncomfortable pose.

When it becomes impossible to feign further interest or face another cup of the Mayor's wine we leave, thinking that Monsieur Vesti is a *très bon* chap and he would get our vote anytime! His next 'orgy' is not until July 21st and we may not be here. That's disappointing!

July 4th

Local radio tells of rain at Wimbledon for the tennis and that French lorry drivers in protest, are blockading the main routes from the ferries, which is affecting holiday makers. We are expecting Paul and Sally and the two boys in a few days time so we are a little apprehensive, as they are driving down via Calais.

It is a surprise to see three American naval ships in the bay, dressed overall with flags in honour of Independence Day. A few sailors are ashore, so we ask one whether there are going to be any special celebrations. "'Fraid not Ma'am, but I guess the town has fireworks tomorrow night." That should be good we thought.

Calling at the butcher's, I order our steak haché in passable French. Standing at my side is another American who is loudly complaining to the butcher that "It's about time you lot learnt to speak English." Whether the butcher understood is uncertain, but it made a few heads turn. At night the US naval ships had replaced their flags with fairy lights which reflect and twinkle in the water through the driving rain, the sound of which almost blots out the accordionist's attempt to find his missed notes.

The following night, the fireworks timed for 10.30pm went off at 9.40pm and by the time we had dashed up to a good viewpoint, it was all over. Either the advertisement was wrong or the officials had decided that, since it is a cloudy night, "Let's get it over with and go home."

July 6th

Cycling into Beaulieu whilst Sam has a siesta, I first call at the bank for a very long wait for some money. The young teller is still learning about the caprices of his computer and repeatedly presses the wrong key, then he has to call the girl with a twitch three times to come and sort him out.

The main purpose for me today is to make a few quick sketches of the trendy sculptures in the park. There is the nude male figure painfully impaled on crossed poles, entwined and undefined male and female figures are left to the imagination, an ugly emaciated male sits in constipated mode on a trestle, and beside a tall green mystery figure is a furtive looking man with a cigarette. The bronze cigarette has been substituted with a dog end by some wag, although it could be just a piece of paper but I dare not touch in case I am blamed for it. There are others too but my progress is hampered by the interest shown by onlookers, which I find too embarrassing so put away my pad and try to memorise the rest of the sculptures.

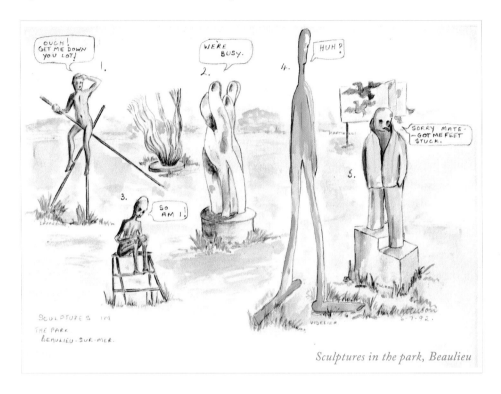

Sculptures in the park, Beaulieu

On the way back I meet an English lady with a dog called Champers and I must listen to a long discourse on the problems of the port and its toilet facilities, and some interesting facts about the Portuguese man 'o war jellyfish. Seemingly a spate of them occur every four years so the sea has to be purified, and as this is now the fourth year that is why we can see the port's clean up boat, not only scooping up the rubbish but jetting disinfectant with a high pressure hose. All this is instigated by the Mayor's insistence on clean beaches. That man certainly has some clout!

To try and get a word in myself, I am tempted to ask her what the town's attitude is towards dogs fouling the pavements, but Champers begins to tug on his lead – he probably read my thoughts.

On arriving back there is an obnoxious stench and much activity outside one of the restaurants, men are scrubbing and hosing the pavement. We learn later that the drains had backed up – an occurrence endemic to this region. Heavily disguised in perfume, it is business as usual that evening and the strains of *Lara's Song* and *Roll out the Barrel* drift across the water as the regular accordionist gropes his way round the notes.

July 9th

The last two days have been spent shopping, cleaning and packing up two holdalls of surplus clothing and books to take to the car for storage in order to make more space on board. Ever since Sam found that length of rope and a useful piece of teak, he does an evening circuit of the waste bins in hope of more treasures.

Paul, Sally, Tom - now ten years old - and Russ, eight, arrive by car, tired and excited, bringing with them much clobber as well as a sail board and fishing tackle.

July 10th

Of course we are up early! With good timing we take the car up to Monaco in time for them to see the changing of the guard at the palace. Outside the Oceanography museum, the boys think it is cool to pose against the model Yellow Submarine. We drive up to Eze for lunch and ice cream, back to the beach, windsurfing, fishing and more ice cream. It is all quite tiring trying to keep up with the energies of youngsters but, at least this year, they are not kicking the heads off the flowers.

We are asked to move the two cars from the square up into the car park over looking the harbour, and within sight. A marquee, with staging and chairs is being erected in the square, "Aha, another of the Mayor's parties?" Not so. It is for the rather posh wedding of the daughter of the president of an eminent airline, which is followed by an outrageous fashion show. All good spectator sport!

July 12th

Today we plan to sail to Antibes but first of all, go up to check on the cars. "Oh no!" Ours has been broken into again, all our clothing and bags have gone, the door lock is sprained and the steering wheel lock is damaged. Words cannot express how cross and upset we feel, especially as the family are here on holiday. Vaguely, we recall two well suntanned fellows leaning over the balustrade when they had finished hawking their 'Rolex' watches the night before, but who knows?

However, we must save the day, and whilst Paul and Sam take the car to the garage Tom and I report to the Gendarmerie and have the letter typed for the insurers, which is now a well practiced ritual. Sally and Russ are left to play on the beach until all that is possible has been dealt with, so we cast off the lines to sail round the corner to anchor in the bay at Villefranche for lunch and a swim.

On mainsail, jib and a lumpy sea, we bounce a further ten miles down to the old harbour at Antibes where Sally makes an instant departure for the Picasso museum. It is agreed that there will be no more mention of the car or missing clothing whilst they are on holiday!

The next few days are spent leisurely revisiting Napoule and St Maxime, anchoring during the day so that each of us can try a hand at windsurfing in the crystal clear water. Going into a marina for the evening is a must due to the promises of ice creams for good behaviour and praiseworthy attempts at helming.

July 17th St Maxime to Port Grimaud

This morning Sam rings the garage and is told that our car will be ready to collect tomorrow. The idea now is to sail just over four miles from St Maxime to Port Grimaud, since it is more accessible for public transport and only a short gentle waft away.

This port is a large and purpose built complex of attractive apartments, many of them having their own moorings. There are shops, bars and restaurants in an intricate system of waterways with many little bridges trying to resemble Venice and needing a map to find the beach. Although there is a ferry boat, we gingerly seat the six of us in the dinghy, which is fine until the outboard engine misbehaves and we have to use the oars to paddle, Indian style for the rest of the way, narrowly missing the No. 6 ferry bus.

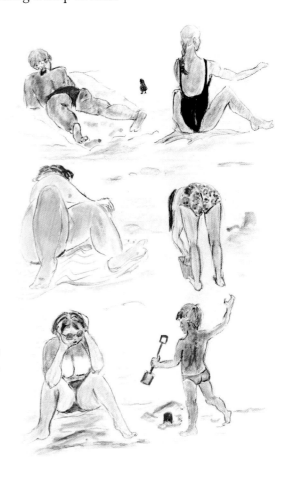

Sam and Paul are up early next day to catch the 9am bus to St Raphael then a train to Beaulieu, where they then have to walk into St Jean to fetch both cars back. What a marathon. Is it really necessary, and just how helpful is it to cope with both a car and a boat? It is a mixed blessing, especially as we are not sure where to park here as the few parking areas there are, all have barriers .

The last few days of their holiday is mainly spent on the beach, in the sea or at the ice cream stalls, and all going to bed exhausted.

Flesh. Beach at Port Grimaud

July 21ˢᵗ

Paul has their car all packed and we bid them a tearful goodbye at 10.30am, leaving us feeling a bit flat and not knowing what to do next. I can't face the laundry and cleaning yet. So, what shall we do? Cycling to the beach we call in at the *Capitainerie* and book another week. We are not in a hurry.

July 23ʳᵈ

95°F is more than hot enough, making every small chore an effort. To try and escape from the heat and do something different, we drive uphill to the old town of Grimaud, where the air is more refreshing. Here are the customary steep steps, narrow winding streets hung with geraniums and an imposing castle. Stunning views from the parapets make the perspiration worth while.

On the way back, we make arrangements at St Tropez marina to leave the car in their park in a few days time, where they assure us it will be safe.

Now we need to cool down, so cycle to the beach to save the embarrassment of the dinghy's dodgy outboard motor, which is tackled the next day. The petrol is sieved through a pop sock and the carburettor is cleaned, which seems to jolly it up considerably. To avoid being drawn into this messy job, I take a bucket to the middle of a quiet little cul-de-sac, up-turn it to sit on and try to paint. By the time I have moved three times for a car to pass, my perspective has gone askew, along with the incentive. Turner never had this problem.

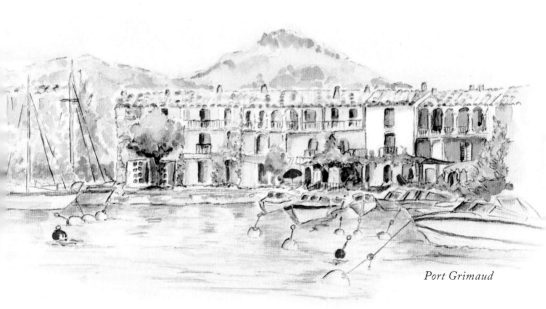

Port Grimaud

The car is taken to St Tropez and parked right outside the office window, but we have no idea how long for. From there, it is easy to take a ferry across back to the boat, and now we can go sailing again. In very humid heat, we idly drift two miles across, anchor off St Tropez for lunch, then three tacks and back into St Maxime marina - not exactly pioneering, but soothing. On nearing our allocated berth, the depth finder panics and shows only seven inches of water under the keel, so we return to Madame *Capitaine* who assures us that it is quite adequate in spite of the eighteen inch range of tide.

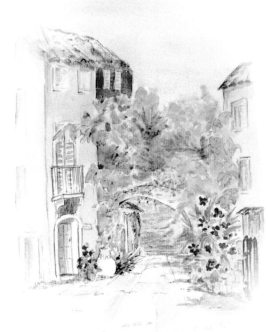

Although we very much like it here, watching the needle matches of boules, the attractive shops and clean beach, after two days, Sam is on edge since listening to the weather report. Strong winds and thunderstorms are expected later, but it does not say how much later.

Port Grimaud

July 29th St Maxime to Cavalaire

Before 9am we are out into a calm sea and have to motor half of the way before there is enough breeze to fill the jib and take us into Cavalaire marina. On cue, the one freak gust of wind comes in time to put the boat broadside onto the pontoon when trying to reverse into a narrow berth. With a little pushing from a nearby crew, it is poked into position and soon we are ready to inspect this resort, being one that we have not been to before. It is quite large and modern, and the beach is well crowded, being towel to towel, toe to jowl situation. Our mats find a small space between the slipway and the dustbin, then we thread a precarious path through the brown basking bodies, and once past the sea edge ball games and frisbies, the water is warm and clear. The marina complex is fairly new and quite attractive with waterside shops and bars, which are not as expensive as expected. The wind and thunder is holding off, there are no arc lamps and no traffic, so we should have a peaceful night. At 10pm, what do we get? Bongo drums!

July 31ˢᵗ

Today we have our first experience in an Aquascope, a catamaran shaped, modernistic craft with a deep central pod enabling you to view the undersea world without getting wet. It cruises out to an obviously regular feeding area teeming with shoals of fish of every shape and colour, and myriads of tiny blue ones darting all around. The only thing that slightly mars this delightful display is the fact that in this confined space, we are sharing it with six other perspiring adults, a baby with sunglasses, comforter, and the over powering need of a nappy change, plus a wet shaggy dog. Whew!

An open air circus in the square is advertised for tonight but starts half an hour late due to a shortage of audience. Well past its use by date, a shaggy Shetland pony staggers round and round the ring on a string for ten minutes, led by a bored youth. This act is followed by the clown throwing his three little boys about, then Madame Katya wobbles round trying to balance on a huge ball. As we quietly leave we notice two moth eaten goats and a dismal donkey patiently awaiting their turn midst their day's droppings. Poor creatures. We are now thinking, just how business-like is it to set out rows of chairs that have to be paid for, but only a few honest citizens do pay and everyone else stands behind the chairs free of charge?

Later we learn that the circus people are paid by the local Mayor or the town council to visit these resorts, so they don't really mind whether they have an audience or not.

August 1ˢᵗ Cavalaire to Lavandou

Our first intention this morning is to catch an early bus to St Tropez to move the car along but on calling at the *Capitainerie* to book another night here, we are told for the first time this year, "You go." It seems that two nights are the limit in this marina and we have already stayed for three. I try a sob story about the car, but he does not relent.

A quick change of plan sees *Kalivala* tacking at six knots under jib and mizzen sails in a brisk breeze, extending the nine miles to thirteen.

In the afternoon we catch the local bus, a smart air conditioned coach driven by a large bossy woman. The car is unscathed, but the purse suffers heavily in spite of some price reduction. Now we need to find another parking place so make enquiries for a lock up garage. Fortunately, we speak to a lady who just so happens to have a space next to her garage and restaurant, which is locked at night. The keys are entrusted to her and we keep our fingers crossed.

Returning hot and tired, a hose down on the pontoon is relaxing but there are new notices on the lamp posts saying *Jazz Festival and Grand Circus*. "Help. They are following us."

The next three days pass pleasantly in Lavandou and at last, the insurance claim is posted - we now know the procedure.

Once again the refrigerator unit is removed, poked, thumped, spoken to roughly and put back again. *Voilà* – we have blast off! To further humour it, the electric fan is put into the under sink cupboard and we have visions of cold drinks and butter that doesn't need spreading with a brush.

In spite of the notice in five languages at the harbour office that *A left place is a lost place*, we take advantage of the light breeze to have a refreshing sail round the bay, taking it in turns to be towed along on the end of a warp to cool off.

Our left place is not lost and the afternoon is spent driving over to Hyères to inspect the facilities and availability. It is not a very attractive port, but it looks useful, is much cheaper and has an adjacent car park. The most sensible option now is to leave the car and return by bus, but apathy takes over in favour of leaving time for an hour on the beach, where there is the search for a square metre of sand to sit on without putting your toe in someone's ear. The *chou-chou* man calls out his wares as he gingerly picks a way between the glistening tanned thighs and bare bosoms with his tray of doughnuts, sandwiches and sugared peanuts. (*Chou-chou*). We don't like crowds, but the cool, clear water is compelling and, *When in Rome...*

Back on the quayside, chickens are being spit roasted, the 'dog bar' has fresh lemon in the water and all is serene, that is until three pop groups belt out their repertoires until early morning, throbbing their drum beats through the hull of the boat, the mattress, pillow and even my deaf ear.

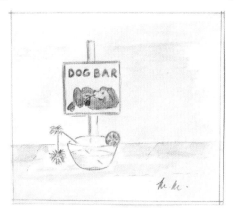
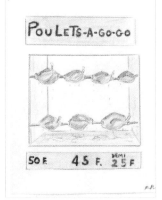

August 5th Lavandou to Hyères

As usual, we leave before the wind has woken up, so have to motor half of the way until lunch time when the engine is turned off to just float freely while we eat. Of course, the wind pipes up about two miles from the destination with the extra gust taking us clumsily onto the Reception Quay. At a third attempt we make a neat landing alongside the wall, only to be asked to move again shortly after, when the wind plays more tricks needing the boat hook to pull us round. A few minutes later we feel less embarrassed when the next yacht to come in, has to be fended off to avoid being blown crossways onto the end of the pontoon. This is closely followed by another craft making a hash of mooring, causing much multi lingual shouting until all boats are secure.

Sam now has time to catch the bus back to Lavandou to fetch the car, the distance being about forty miles by road as opposed to twelve and a half nautical miles by sea. While he is away, I explore to find that all the useful shops are at hand, as are the waterfront bars, bistros, and crowded beach. The town is not greatly attractive, but we shall be able to see the car about ten yards from the boat.

Today we have done much plugging in, unplugging and coiling, re-plugging the electrics, and unfurling and furling hose pipes and warps so are looking forward to our bed. There are no security lights shining down the hatch, but what can we hear? The regular comings and goings of the ferry to the islands of Port Cros and Porquerolle, the aircraft coming to land at the Turin/Hyeres airport behind us and a Beatles serenade percolating through between.

August 7th Hyères

Having a car can be a nuisance one day and a blessing the next, but it does enable you to see much more of the surroundings. It is an interesting drive down the peninsula of Presqu'ile de Giens, where there is the sea on one side and the lakes and salt pans on the other. This is a bird spotter's paradise where flocks of little plovers and tern mingle with the wading avocets, heron and, best of all the flamingos. They are not as pink as usual, but do have the characteristic bright pink, wing flash. From the small port on the tip of this flat strip of land, ferries ply across to Isle de Porquerolles, where we hope to visit again. This area is more interesting than first thought, making today a bonus to have the car.

Because it is marginally cheaper here, we pay for two more nights and drive up to the old town of Hyères, which is a few miles inland. This too has its surprises as we climb ever upwards through the narrow old streets. If we have translated a local lady correctly when she gives us a long historical account, it is believed that St Claire's Chateau is where the man who discovered the *Venus de Milo* lived and died. The castle is now closed but in a high wall, a worm eaten old door creaks open onto a lovely garden with archways, vivid flowers, bushes, swallow-tailed butterflies and a balustrade overlooking the whole peninsula beyond the red pantiles of the town. Back down the alleys, a cool beer is welcome before sitting on the steps of the twelfth century Church of the Templars to eat a slab of quiche.

Another change of plan. We drive into St Mandrier to ask about parking and are lucky to find an excellent lock up garage, but to leave it today and have to return by catching a ferry and four different buses is just too daunting, so we drive back instead. In our absence, the barometer has taken a dramatic dive and an evil smell emanates from the refrigerator. What is it this time? Just the milk turning into cheese again.

Tonight, the strains of Elvis Presley filter across from a bar, but not far enough away.

August 9ᵗʰ

Although the day starts with hot sunshine, the forecast is for thunderstorms, hail and high winds, with the same again tomorrow – just when we intend to move on. By 11am the sea is choppy and a boat comes in reporting force six winds between here and Porquerolle. Being curious to look at the sea state, we go down to the harbour wall and are shocked to see a very small motor boat floundering in the heavy waves and in it are two men, a small boy and a dog. Their engine has failed, one man is shouting and waving frantically, and whilst the other tries to fend it off the rocks with a boat hook, the boy cries and the dog barks fiercely. Quickly, I run back to call up the *Capitaine* on Channel 9. I am not sure if he understands my emergency call in fractured French, and I certainly cannot translate his reply, but a helpful man on the next boat relays the message and very soon a dinghy with an outboard engine reaches the terrified trio, followed by the harbour launch which tows them to safety. Not so lucky is the poor exhausted young seagull with both wings broken, which has no chance of rescue as it is dashed against the rocks out of our reach.

The weather men are right. At 7pm an advancing large black cloud obliterates the sun and gives the best thunderstorm since Florida. Only just in time do we close the hatches before the torrential rain and hail strikes, accompanied by a non stop display of impressive lightning. Sam sits entranced, watching the wind speed indicator swing from twenty knots to forty-five as it gusts, and rates it better than television. When the worst of the rain has passed through, we watch the continuing spectacular lightning reflecting over the sea which is now glassy calm since the wind dropped. For an evening's entertainment, it makes a change from pop music.

August 11ᵗʰ Hyères to Porquerolles – and return

A bicycle tyre punctures on the way for the shopping in readiness for the island trip, but we are still ready to leave at 9am. There is a frisky breeze and a slightly choppy sea – that is until we reach the gap between the mainland and the island. As if a door has opened suddenly, the breeze is a strong wind, the chop builds up into sizeable waves and our only picture falls off the wall. Clothes pegs and kettle are stowed in the oven - its door tied shut with a belt. On trying to ring Porquerolles marina to ask for a berth, it seems that many others are doing the same and we cannot make contact, so keep going and arrive in the marina to be told, "Marina full. Go and anchor outside." The anchorage is also full, and a force 7 wind has just been broadcast on the radio. The choice now is to head into the wind for another ten miles, or return to Hyères when that port might also now be full.

Cowardice rules. We turn back to enjoy an exhilarating sail under a reduced jib at a speed of six knots, to find that our berth on number nine pontoon has already been taken. The *Capitainerie* is closed until three o'clock. We are told to go and anchor.

A little pleading allows us to remain on the reception quay until that magic hour when the *Capitaine* returns from his three hour lunch break and siesta. It takes almost an hour in his office before a berth is allocated, as he is throwing a wobbly and threatens to close the office and the harbour because there are too many boats, and it is all getting a bit too much for him.

What a berth he gives us. No. 100 is in a tight corner, blocked by a large power boat that has an over hanging dinghy on its davits, and another power boat trailing a dinghy near a large white mooring buoy. A bit of shouting brings attention from one of the owners who kindly moves further forward, re-positions his dinghy, then helps to nudge us into the corner.

I suppose we should be grateful to have been found any berth at all, even if it is opposite the piano bar.

August 12th Hyères to St Mandrier
The sun on a fly-past of a flock of flamingos is a fine sight early this morning when on the way to the port office for a weather report. It is not too promising, but it makes no difference – we have been evicted! "Six nights is over the limit," we are told.

Leaving at 9am, we have to motor for six miles until past Porquerolle where the sea is still rather disturbed off the headlands, then we can let out the jib for the last seven miles. Now we need to locate the buoys called, The 'Two Brothers' which warn of the rocks at the turn towards Toulon. After much scouring of the coastline through the binoculars, what we thought was a fisherman in a red shirt, standing up in a little boat ultimately reveals himself to be one of the 'Brothers' - the red marker buoy we are looking for. A few moments later, a man in a green shirt also comes into view.

Just before the entrance to St Mandrier lies the forbidding looking destroyer together with other neglected old naval hardware that is remembered from the last brief visit. Once inside the small sheltered marina, there is the pleasant little town, no arc lights, no piano bar, and no bongo drums just the sound of the fenders having an occasional squeak.

As we are supposed to be crossing the Atlantic with Carl in November, leaving from Bandol, we must find somewhere to winter our boat, and make phone calls to a few marinas. La Ciotat cannot accommodate us and Bandol can only give us four months, so although it is small and further east than wished, we try the *chantier* here. They are most obliging, almost welcoming and are very much cheaper but for some reason, we have to book it for a whole year out of the water on hard standing. It is also arranged that we can stay on our berth until August 26th as long as we pay now. We pay and stay!

Chapter 8

Spiced Loaf

Between mistrals, thunderstorms and sunshine we take interest in the frequent events, or manifestations in the town's Programme of Events. On the harbour side is a market, the tantalising aroma of spit roasting chickens lures us into the midst of all the bowls of olives, black, green, stuffed, un-stuffed, herbed and garlicked, the rolls of Provence material, flowers and shrubs. Alongside hop the live rabbits, hens, canaries and pigeons, clawing and scratching to be free of their tiny cages.

Further down in the square are rows of chairs and platforms being erected in readiness for some event – a Mayor's party perhaps? Continuing our exploratory bike ride, a Franco-Italian cemetery is at the top of a steep hill and has a fine outlook across the sea – most cemeteries seem to have the best views. The return route passes the harbour, and we see that the 'event' is already in progress, it is *Les Joutes* or water jousting, so we take a grandstand seat nearest to the action to watch the antics.

There are two, long, painted wooden boats - one red, one blue, with a cantilevered platform sloping up from the stern. The contestants, in team colours wear a chest pad and wooden shield, the left hand holds a sectioned box to fend off with, and the right hand wields a long pole. When they are suitably poised on the top of the platform, the two boats row towards each other at a steady pace, approaching port side to port side, ship their oars, and the two opponents lift their poles, lunge forward to poke into the box-like shield in the attempt to topple each other into the water.

Sometimes one is down at the first poke but usually, there is a hard struggle with much jeering and cheering from the stands. The winner then takes his bow and poses like a toreador, and the loser has to swim back. The junior team, age between twelve and sixteen years old, and have learnt the triumphal pose already. Men of all ages take part but are mostly young machos with the physique of a rugby full back, and come by coach from as far away as Marseilles and the Rhone river for this three day event. Today it is the quarter finals of the Annual Contests of Water Jousting.

In the morning we had decided to fetch the car from Toulon, it is so beautiful that I change Sam's mind for him and we sail to the island of Embiez instead. After thirteen miles of easy sailing, we come to very high, forbidding cliffs topped with an old semaphore and ancient fortifications near the rocky approach to the harbour. The entrance is well buoyed, and there is no problem obtaining a berth for £10 per night.

There are many woodland walks, little bays, a few small shops and a museum in a garden setting. A little white tourist train chugs and hoots as it winds round past the very new church which still smells fresh plaster, but is a bit

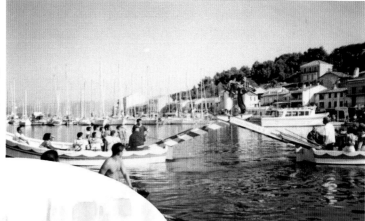

Les Joutes, St Mandrier

spoilt by the seating – white plastic patio chairs. The island also has its own bank, which resembles a broom cupboard with a safe in the corner, and is staffed by a spotty, gum chewing girl wearing a T-shirt over a swim suit and an indifferent young man in baggy shorts. A visit to the aquarium is a bit disappointing after Sea world in Florida.

The whole island and its facilities, belong to Paul Ricard, of aperitif fame, who also owns the car racing track at Castellet on the mainland.

After spending two more days, we are quite sorry to leave this comparatively unspoilt little haven. On the tranquil sail back to St Mandrier, the 'Two Brothers' buoys are not mistaken for the men in little boats and we are back in our berth well in time to catch the Sit-Cat ferry across the bay to Toulon. This fast craft conveniently lands adjacent to the pedestrianised old part of the town, which has parks, gardens and fountains, all much more attractive than anticipated, so we take time to look around on the walk to the garage. Outside one of the many, many shoe shops, an old man with a rickety wooden street organ churns out unrecognisable tunes opposite the music shop, which is trying to drown him out with *A Whiter Shade of Pale*.

The car is intact and we drive back to St Mandrier without getting lost. Each day seems to have some kind of entertainment. A Marionette Show is advertised one evening in the square, where a full-sized stage has been erected. The ragged curtains draw back to reveal a booth the size of a Punch and Judy show, and that is what it is, except that *Guinol* is the French equivalent of Punch but lacks the crocodile, policeman and sausages.

During the mornings, there are jobs to be done to prepare the boat for winter. Fuel is emptied from the outboard motor and the little generator and cupboards are cleaned. After doing some useful work, we can take even more exercise in the *Foret Communale*, which has a laid out *Route Sportif* alongside the paths. This is a kind of assault course where every hundred metres there is a notice board to tell you what to do – press-ups, stretching etc. There are parallel bars, balancing bars, bars to swing on or jump over, but no refreshment bars. No wonder the cemetery is adjacent.

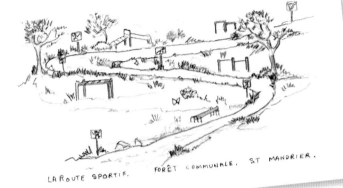

LA ROUTE SPORTIF.   FORÊT COMMUNALE. ST MANDRIER.

What a surprise – the circus is in town. We must see this, it is a different family. Set up in the square, the majority of spectators stand behind the chairs and only a few pay for seats, as usual. First there is the poor pony being led round on a string, but this is different. Two little girls come on and hold a pole two feet off the ground, then when the pony reaches it they lower it right down for it to step over. Next is the young man performing hand stands on a pile of chairs, then a very wobbly tight-rope walker staggers across the ring barely two feet off the ground, whilst the father balances his two coquettish girls, one on each hand. Just as we are beginning to wonder if this can get any more exciting, on comes the ugliest brown dog I have ever seen, to begrudgingly climb a short ladder, teeter across a plank and jump through a hoop. It's lopsided frayed frill round its neck does nothing to enhance its image, which looks like an unfortunate liaison between a scruffy poodle and a miserable monkey. Just after half time, a stage hand dressed as a clown, is noisily stacking the spare chairs and fencing into a van – perhaps ready for a quick get a way. The audience, however, has been wildly appreciative throughout, which sets us thinking – is it because we have become too old, too sophisticated and spoilt by television to be able to fully enjoy the naivety and simplicity of a struggling family tradition? Or is it really just rubbish and exploitation?

Between short bursts of sorting out old books, nests of plastic bags and other clutter under the sink, (where did that putrefied carrot come from?)we enjoy being interrupted by other cruising neighbours. A beer on the boat from Poole, a glass of wine on the yacht from Plymouth, and Pastis on the King's Lynn craft – not all on the same day of course, and then it is our turn to be the hosts, so the days pass quickly by.

The *Capitaine* tells us that, because we shall be here for more than six months, French bureaucracy states that we must again have a form from the Customs office with an official stamp. That office is closed, so we must go to La Seyne, a few miles away. Arriving at the address given that too is closed. Try another office, also closed! The tourist office should know. The charming girl there gives more directions, which also prove to be wrong. With the help of a passer-by, the right office is located, which just happens to be straight across the road from the tourist office. I could not resist going back to show her. Here they politely apologise that they do not have the necessary forms and that we must go into Toulon. By now we are hot, tired, and just a little out of humour, as we drive to the next given address, which again is wrong. But we are getting close. It is next door upstairs where, in less than five minutes, a form is filled in, rubber stamped, and the customs' men are happy. In spite of all the hassle and inconvenience, everyone has been most courteous and helpful.

A few wrong turns in Toulon puts us on an interesting route through an underground car park and along a disused railway track.

In our absence a platform has been erected at the end of our pontoon – please don't let it be a rock festival.

August 24th St Mandrier

Another message filters through from Carl, a request to visit his boat, *Hope II* which is still in Bandol. It seems a good idea to take our oilskins and sleeping bags with us in readiness for the Atlantic crossing when we return in November. Carl's new wife is amiable and together we make a few constructive ideas for victualling, and some vague plans for the passage. She is apprehensive about the trip and so am I, especially as there are still problems with the plumbing. Into the car we load a large box of Carl's equipment, the log and depth finder to be taken back to England and be serviced. We are ready to leave at 6.30pm. It is a pleasant drive back, but we are tired and only wish for a quick supper, bed, and a quiet night. No chance. There is a wedding party in the rooms beneath the *Capitanerie*, where the disco beats and the nuptials revel until early morning.

August 25th

There is now only one full day left before leaving again for home. The bimini is taken down, outboard engine and sails stowed, purifier put into the water tank, plus many other last minute chores. A welcome interruption is given by the large *Grand Banks* power boat noisily entering the marina and making a worse mess of reversing than us. At third attempt into different berths he finally succeeds, comes down from his upper control deck, struts boldly along the lower deck and makes a flourishing bow to applause from a gathering of interested onlookers.

The car, now proving to be worth its presence is filled beyond capacity with surplus fenders, warps, spare clothing, and the ladder that was rescued from the sea bed.

It is a bad decision to stay in our berth tonight instead of mooring at the boatyard ready for lift out tomorrow, as we later find out what the staging is for – another disco.

August 26th St Mandrier to Hamble

An early start today moving to the boatyard at 8.30am as arranged, only to hear that the workmen now prefer to lift out the boat after lunch instead. Only a few moments of wheedling in our best school French is needed to change their minds for them, and within an hour *Kalivala* is lifted, pressure-hosed, chocked up in a cradle on the back row, and hopefully well sheltered until our return in November.

Farewell to St Mandrier, the *Capitaine* and the friends we have made, we are on our way home.

Driving through stunning mountain scenery via Ollioules, Aix en Provence, Arles and Nîmes, we reach a small, pretty auberge in Florac at 6.30pm. The evening meal is excellent, the adequate bedroom is … er … quaint, unique, different? The assured en-suite consists of a wash basin in the corner and a bidet on wheels, which swings out on a flexible hose behind a wooden screen. Not exactly *très chic*, but it makes us chuckle before spending the night clawing the way back from the middle of the sagging bed.

The next night in Lussac, I test the bed with the proprietress, bouncing on it together before making the booking. The dustbin men start work at 4.30am here.

The ferry from Ouistreham to Portsmouth leaves at 4.30 pm. The sea is rough and the French waiter in the cafeteria throws a very Gallic tantrum over the platefuls of abandoned food as he steps gingerly over the prostrate bodies on the floor – poor things.

The ship docks at 10.30pm and within half an hour we are home in Hamble, a comfortable bed and apart from the owls, no night noises. What luxury!

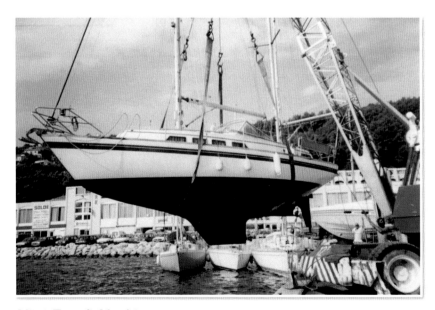

Mise à Terre, St Mandrier

Chapter 9

Grouse simmered in Port

For the last month we have been enjoying seeing family and friends and making endless trips to the local tip with the garden cuttings. Then a phone call from Carl, who requests that we return to Bandol as soon as possible. He wishes to have a shakedown cruise to Corsica and Sardinia via St Tropez, before leaving in November in company of other boats crossing the Atlantic to celebrate the centenary of Christopher Columbus' voyage. This all sounds most exciting, although we are a little apprehensive of possible personality clashes.

This sudden summons causes a flurry of visits to the dentist, barber, hairdresser and the doctors' surgery for injections against Tetanus and Hepatitis, and sugar lumps for Poliomyelitis, before being ready to fly back on the 8th of October – a month earlier than anticipated.

The aggravation begins at the airport when Sam expresses his wish that Carl's repaired electronic equipment should not be x-rayed; he has to be convinced that the x-ray will not harm it. Our cabin baggage is too heavy, then I remember that our third injection for Hepatitis has to be kept refrigerated and it is in the bag that is now trundling across to the aircraft! The response to my tale of woe is a frosty, "Unless Madame wants to delay take off". 'Madame didn't – but as it happens, we are delayed for forty minutes anyway.

Landing at Marseilles we are met by an employee from the La Ciotat plant, and first taken to the offices where we impatiently sit waiting for three hours while Carl finishes his business talk, before taking us over to Bandol to his boat, *Hope II*.

There we are introduced to two other prospective crew members, Janine and Pierre, both very pleasant but they speak only very little English. Also we meet young Nigel, who is employed as a boat-minder come engineer. As we now are well aware, the electrics on this boat are fickle, which tends to sap your confidence in the electric flushing system in the heads.

Everyone retires to bed early, for tomorrow we are sailing to St Tropez again to see the annual racing events of the Nioulargue.

October 10th Bandol to St Tropez

At 5am there are stirrings below, which we try to ignore. But at 6am the engine starts and it is impossible to ignore it any longer. I emerge in time to take in and stow the heavy, almost life-sized fenders as we leave the marina.

The sea is grey with a hefty swell, and the struggling sun surrenders to a rain cloud as we sail along with a small foresail, reefed main and mizzen sails.

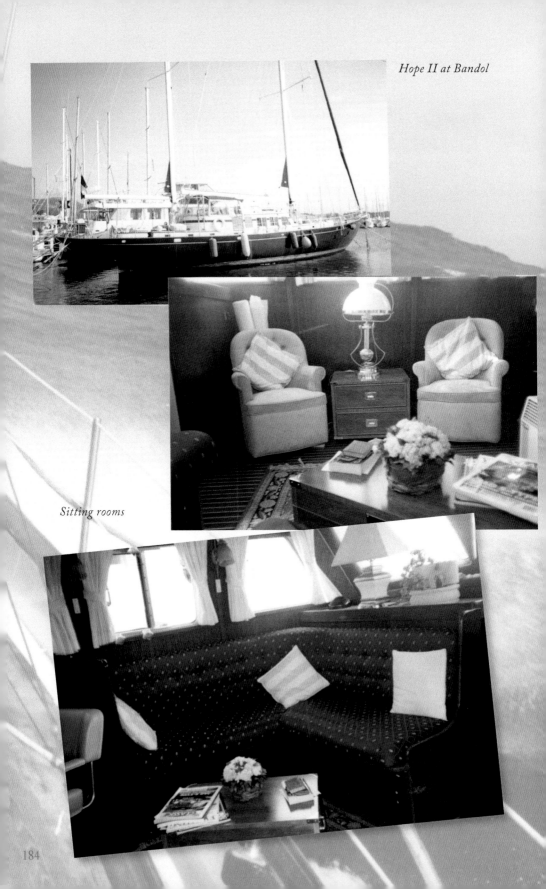

Hope II at Bandol

Sitting rooms

184

Below deck I find that nothing has been stowed and am just in time to catch a cut glass vase of two dozen red roses before it hits the floor. Underneath the cushions I wedge two of the free standing table lamps, before the third one falls over at the same time as the huge silk flower arrangement! How very unseaman-like.

Carl is at the helm, Sam and Nigel are in the bilges discussing electric wiring, whilst I join Janine in a keep fit class that Bella is instructing, but within an hour the two girls have succumbed to sea-sickness, missing lunch and the rest of the afternoon. These are to be our Atlantic crew mates?

Passing the 'Two Brothers' rocks off St Mandrier, we think of *Kalivala* and hope that all is well with her.

On nearing St Tropez, it is a wonderful sight to see the fleet of large schooners, some three-masted, all in full sail, racing towards the finish line. Anchoring off the heliport, we can sit and watch this fine spectacle, making it well worth the sixty-mile passage.

A loud bang wakes everyone up at 2am to see a large catamaran swinging onto us on the change of tide. The ladies go back to bed while the menfolk re-anchor . The morning reveals just a small bruise on the strake, but a big bruise to the skipper's pride.

October 11ᵗʰ

Ashore, two hours are spent paying homage to some of the beautiful classic yachts in the old harbour, which include the 1930's J Class *Endeavour*, *Attaria*, *Merit*, *Mirabelle*, *Flica* and Eric Taberly's famous *Pen Duik*.

Carl then insists on buying us all a navy blue polo shirt with a white collar and has the boat name *Hope II* embroidered on it. The shop does not have an extra small one for me, so mine is six inches too large in every direction, and not exactly chic in St Tropez. Janine kindly offers to shorten it, but that still won't solve the sleeves and girth.

For suppressed entertainment, this evening we spend an hour watching Carl and Bella searching for the source of some moth grubs seen on the galley ceiling. A loud oath and a scream heralds the finding of a seething nest of the B***** critters in a box of porridge oats which has been left since the previous Transatlantic crossing over a year ago. Chaos ensues as packets of cereal, flour, biscuits, lentils and coffee from all the cupboards are angrily thrown across the floor, for someone else to brush up and dispose of.

October 12ᵗʰ

Like a factory hooter the electric loos sound their alarm at 5am. Sam gets up, I turn over, but when I emerge later, there is no coffee left and I cannot make any because for some reason, when there is no shore power, it needs the generator to work the coffee maker, cooker and microwave oven.

Motoring in a calm sea, we are now on our way back to Bandol. The men are still discussing electrics, whilst the ladies take the sun on the foredeck.

Nigel is looking very worried, he has re-fixed the depth finder and we suspect that he has put something in back to front.

Early the next morning, Carl and Bella leave for the airport, as she is going back to America for two weeks and I am to be left in charge of domestics and feeding three men. 'Help! What is going on? I thought we were sailing to Corsica.'

In order to have a bathroom en suite, instead of one opposite with a dripping shower, we persuade Nigel to change with us. He is not well pleased, but at least he now has more space. Sam helps him with the boat work, and I set about preparing supper. I am not enamoured with the difficulties in this galley, as being only five feet two inches tall, I cannot reach things and have to climb up onto the sink top every few minutes to search for items in the cupboards, and the electric hobs are slow to respond. Carl does not arrive back until 8.15pm, by which time supper has been re-heated three times, but at least he eats it. Some days he is much later and has already eaten, or insists that we eat out with no prior warning, then I am more than a little peeved as I don't like cooking that much.

Why is there no mention of Corsica or Sardinia? No plans are being made for any voyages, and we dare not ask.

The days go by. Most mornings Sam now puts on a tie and goes, by request, with Carl to the La Ciotat office, leaving me with Nigel who lounges on the settee watching the television until 10.30am, when he goes for a shower, leaving me to clear away his dirty breakfast dishes. (Bite your tongue, Monica.) He has been assigned to paint Carl and Bella's newly acquired flat in Cassis, but manages to apply a mixture of both satin and matt emulsion to the kitchen, whereupon Carl lets everyone hear his raging displeasure.

When I am left alone on the boat I promise myself a peaceful day, but before long I find that I am exorcising some of my building resentment by polishing the stainless steel refrigerator, the chart table and floors, then hoovering, washing and ironing - and I don't like housework!

A swarm of tiny wine flies come in to the saloon at the same time as an ominous gurgling sound comes from the bathroom where the stinking, over-full holding tank is regurgitating across our bathroom floor. I do know that it has to be pumped out from somewhere in the bowels of the engine room and I think I know how. First, you need to grope around with a torch to find the light switch to reveal an area the size of our dining room. Then take a long steel rod and insert it into a hole on the floor but, there are six holes to choose from. Picking the nearest hole I flick a switch and listen for the gurgling sound – silence. Second time lucky, and now there is just the two bathroom floors to wash and disinfect, and meanwhile there has been another invasion of wine flies. It is then that I have an overwhelming desire to kick Carl's expensive, teak coffee table, yet with much willpower I restrain myself – but may God forgive me for my uncharitable thoughts. I think I am beginning to understand vandalism and its causes.

I tell myself yet again that many people would be envious of this lifestyle, living in the South of France on an 86ft luxury yacht with all expenses paid. Yes, we are privileged, but would still rather be doing our own thing than be beholden to someone.

The arrival of a young, personable electrician from our home town is welcome, except that I now have another man to feed. Soon there are wires and cables to trip over, and the transducer for the depth finder is found to be broken in half, so Nigel is sent up the mast a few times and succeeds in wiring the radio antenna to the Loran Direction finder. Stupid boy!

In spite of all my efforts to keep his boat clean, Carl still stamps around shouting, "I can't stand filth," and then complains that his stomach is off, so drinks two glasses of orange juice and a bottle of beer, then declines my spaghetti bolognese. So my tongue is bitten again!

With the Loran, transducer and all other electrics now trustworthy, the real electrician flies back home - perhaps some plans can now be made, as we are becoming impatient and very unhappy with this situation. Carl and Bella are now engrossed with furnishing their new flat, and there is still no mention of sailing.

October 29th

Whilst crunching our cornflakes this morning the subject of our return flight tickets arises, and we realise just how much we want to escape from this unpredictable waiting game as we can only foresee more aggravation. "Oh, heck. They expire today!" Panic.

Sam goes to the office with Carl as usual, whist I hastily pack our bags and wait for Sam to return. Bella and Nigel are more than a little surprised when they surface from their respective beds just before 11am, especially as they will now have to make their own meals and wash up.

Just as I am beginning to worry if Carl will let Sam go, he arrives back at 11.30am and a sulky Nigel drives us into Marseilles airport. What a wonderful feeling of freedom – no more ruined meals, no regurgitating drains, no tenterhooks or lazy deckhand. But what a waste of three weeks. The relief is so euphoric that for the first time, we eat all of the plastic airline lunch.

November 13th A second helping of grouse

At Carl's bidding, and with high hopes we are once more on our way to Bandol. Is this, at last, for the grand crossing? The sun rises into a clear blue sky, and the fields are sifted with icing sugar frost as the taxi drives to the airport, and there is a feeling of excitement, even though it is Friday the thirteenth. The excitement doesn't last for long though!

Within three days, we are back to the old routine of Sam to the office, Bella out to ballet classes, neck massage, manicures, dentist, facials and exercise classes, while I battle with the domestics and the obnoxious overflows. Luckily, the cause is later found to be due to over filling the freshwater tank, which then drains into the grey water tank, which is obviously not adequate. Thankfully, Nigel has now been dispensed with.

Each day I try to take a brisk walk as an escape, and come across a small sheltered cove where, even in November it is warm enough to join other sunbathers among the mounds of sea grass where the little pied wagtails scavenge like clockwork toys.

Outside the cove, the sea is bashing on the rocks and throwing stones across the road. By five o'clock, it suddenly becomes very cold and one day the heater would not work, so now what is wrong? Tracing the flex back to the source of shore power, I find the plug hanging down in the water, then draped over the mooring lines of the adjacent boat, just out of reach. The rough sea had jerked it out of the socket .

A few contortions and just short of falling head first into the murky marina, it is hauled back, and I remember to dry it before slackening the cable and plugging back in. I do not care for the responsibility of being left alone in charge of someone else's dish washer, washing machine, microwave oven, untrustworthy deep freezer and rubbish plumbing.

Come the weekend, Carl and Sam are taking their pleasure in the bilges, from where much flushing, sucking and gurgling is heard and an obnoxious pong permeates throughout the whole boat. Taps, sinks and loos cannot be used until they have satisfied themselves that what appeared to be a blockage, has been cleared.

Bella and I had escaped to the butcher's, but just as she begins to prepare a rather complicated stew, she remembers that she has to collect her cleaning lady for the flat. Good excuse I thought, as she leaves me with a mound of meat and vegetables and a recipe written in Spanish. When I have chopped everything up she returns, gives me a few vague instructions before dashing off to Marseilles with Carl to shop for an evening dress for their trip to Paris next week. "What? It is the first we've heard of this. I can't believe it. What are we here for, cheap labour?

A walk along the cliff path to watch the rough sea breaking over the rocks helps to quell our uncharitable thoughts as we muse on the fading likelihood of this Atlantic jaunt. On our return, Bella has supposedly been smitten with some kind of allergy and retires to bed, once again leaving me with the huge pan of continental concoction. Tentatively, I have to disturb her to ask whether this is meant to be soup in a bowl or a knife and fork job. This hearty soup tastes better than it looks, but I do wonder what will happen to the remaining gallon?

November 25th
Carl and Bella have left for Paris, and in spite of the annoyance, we feel to be on holiday and Sam doesn't go to the office. Instead, we take the little company car to drive over to St Mandrier to see *Kalivala*. All is clean and dry below; it feels so cosy and homely compared to *Hope II* that we long to stay,

but sadly close up the hatches again to drive up to the Corniche Spectaculaire and along to the forest near Six Fours, where we park the car.

It is a lovely walk up to an ancient chapel where there are breathtaking views from both sides of a peninsula, to the bay of Toulon on one side and across to Sanary, Bandol and beyond La Ciotat on the other. We are really enjoying this day without obligations.

Needing some provisions, we stop on the way back to collect a few items – but where is my money? My purse is empty, all credit cards gone together with the £35 sterling for the taxi home. "Not again?" So carefully had I stowed my handbag under the seat and covered it over before locking the car, yet nothing appears to have been disturbed. Miserable and cross with ourselves, we return our purchases and make yet another visit to the Gendarmerie where, with a few Gallic shrugs, the familiar insurance claim is thumped out with boredom and one finger on an antique typewriter. The gendarme has seen it all before and so have we. By now we should be more streetwise – and we thought we were having an enjoyable day.

November 27th

It is a lovely warm day, and still feeling in holiday mood we suddenly decide to go to the Ile de Bendor, just a few miles offshore from Bandol. The 11am ferry is delayed a while due to the delivery of the island's Christmas trees. (Goodness, is it that near already?) Three men engage in comic antics as they try to remove the trees from the lorry where they have become entangled. After much pulling, pushing, shouting and cracking of branches, they are duly dragged onto the ferry ramp, and the onset of the festive spirit sets off for the seven-minute crossing .

Bendor is small, quite attractive, and also owned by Paul Ricard, the same as Embiez. Whilst walking its circumference and spending ten minutes in the Wine Museum, we encounter only five other people; it seems that Embiez is closed for the winter, so in just over an hour we are ready for the return ferry. This leaves enough time to visit the La Ciotat office for Sam to check that all is in order during Carl's absence.

Normally I say that I never become bored when I am alone, but now, on my knees polishing the floor on this boat, my eyes begin to prickle. "Why am I doing this?"

Carl is a very high powered business man with anxieties, a new wife and homes, so do not like to ask about the situation for fear of causing an atmosphere. We must hang in there, wait – and just enjoy France!

December 4th Glazed pear

What now? Carl is expecting a prospective buyer for *Hope II*, so more polishing is demanded. A very astute cockney gent delves into every corner asking pertinent questions, and Carl is at his most charming self, while on deck I am mentally willing the man to 'buy it please,' and that would resolve the situation. The rest of the fleet doing the transatlantic crossing must have left by now, so we must stop thinking about it, and it feels quite a relief.

The boat has not been sold, Carl and Bella are going to Spain so we are free again!

Having still got the use of a car, we take the opportunity to look at more of the surrounding area. Set in a pretty valley, Moulin de St Come is an old olive oil press building which now sells regional products such as soap, herbs, preserves, Provence materials, wine and all grades of olive oil, all very attractively displayed at inflated prices.

A short drive from there is Cadiere d'Azure, a slightly down market medieval town which has now closed for lunch, except for a small *boulangerie* where we buy a filled baguette. This is eaten up in the hills, beneath pine trees before reaching the vineyard of Chateau de Pibernon. This is the domain of the wine we have enjoyed several times in a little back street restaurant when taken out by Carl, and where Mama still declares her love for Sam! Madame here speaks very good English, and we have an enlightening tour of vats and barrels before sampling her reds, whites and rosés then buying just two bottles of Pibernon Rouge 1989 at £7 each.

Along a rough and bumpy track is another interesting looking Chateau, so we try that one next, sampling their vintage brew, and buying only one bottle.

"Oh, look! There's another one, and since we are passing, we may as try that too!"

After more mock discernment, the sampling results in buying three cheaper bottles with the dubious name of Loubière. Now well fortified, we return via St Cyr and are surprised to find that police have gated off some of the roads, and traffic is in chaos. Booths are being erected along the waterfront and there is much activity in the market place as a throne-like chair, a large chest and a mound of moth eaten, red velvet curtains are trundled across the road from out of the town hall annexe. Pennants hanging from the trees advertise, Fête du vin de Bandol 1992. So that's what it is all for – more wine!

The next day, the wind is very strong and the waves are crashing onto the rocks. The market place is now transformed into a theatrical scene, with a long table bearing flowers, pumpkins, and candelabra that blow over in the wind. There is a balustrade, statues, rocks, a stage and a huge hairy mask hanging from trees, which we assume represents 'Bacchus' the God of wine.

From the aft deck, we watch large barrels arriving and the booths being decorated with branches, vine leaves and heather. It should be an interesting day tomorrow, and we have no other obligations.

December 6th

More booths have sprung up during the night, these are mainly for food. One of them is right at the end of our gang plank, making our access ashore a tricky obstacle course, but as a reward for tolerance, we are given several slices of prosciutto and a noggin of cheese, which will be appreciated at lunch time.

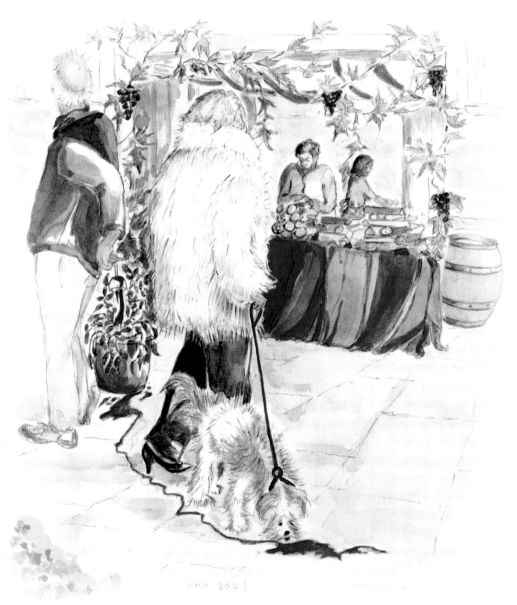

Lap dog

Wine festival Bandol - tipping a few into the bushes

Other stalls are piled high with regional cheeses, hams, muffins tarte tatins, large squares of pizza and quiche, and bread in all shapes.

At 10am a drummer heralds a procession of characters. First comes an impressive Christopher Columbus astride a shaggy old horse, Don Quixote follows with his imbecile servant, then the Royal Court primp by. The King is quite mad, rolls his eyes and makes intermittent short bursts of falsetto singing, whilst his queen is serene and demure in black velvet and her courtesans shiver in their décolletage dresses. The local schoolchildren are all wearing masks as they trot, skip and straggle along behind them.

The Royal entourage then begins to visit each wine booth in turn, and the King extols the virtues of each wine as he samples, rolls his eyes and reaches for a few top notes.

Meanwhile, there are other high standard entertainments, which include the fiery Spanish flamenco dancers, a children's choir, guitarists, modern dances, and literary extracts recited by Don Quixote and his servant.

Sauntering slowly along with our wine glasses, we taste some, drink some, spit some out and also do the same as many others
– tip some into the bushes or flower pots!

Wine festival at Bandol
- never
again!

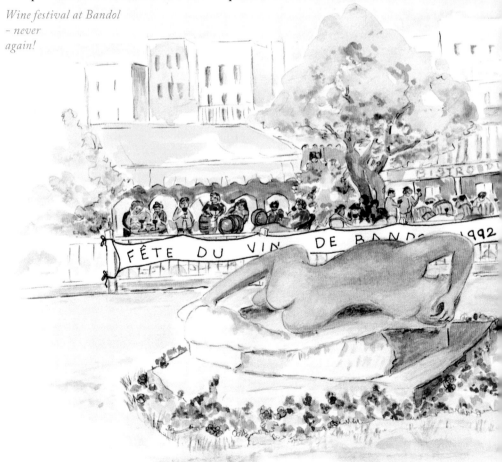

All the vintners are dressed in Spanish costume and make a most picturesque and jolly atmosphere, with no untoward behaviour in spite of the free flowing wine.

At lunchtime, we watch more dancing from on deck then realise that we cannot face an all afternoon session to sample the wines that we missed, so return later just to mingle. Several dishevelled, sturdy horses are pulling barrel wagons round to replenish stock, and the King is still making his visits, spiel and high notes, he must have a very strong constitution.

For some time, I trail after a lady in a very hairy fur coat and her look-alike dog to try to take a photograph, but there are too many people in the way, so I just have to commit her to memory. It has been an unexpected pleasure today, being on the front row for this great French tradition.

Whoever it was, must have worked quickly and quietly all night, as this morning the only signs of yesterday's festivities are a bit of trampled grass and a few red wine stains on the path.

Now all is back to hum-drum norm: Carl and Bella are back, Sam goes to the office, and even the shops are closed on Mondays!

December 9th

A walk to the little sheltered cove of Renecros helps to boost sagging spirits, it is so peaceful here with the warm sun on my face, listening to the gentle lap of the water yet I think it is time we went home. Shall we miss this when we are back in the wet and cold of an English winter? Then come thoughts of a comfortable bed, cupboards I can reach, plumbing that works and people to talk to. What is the best option?

A decision is made, flights are booked in two days time, and there is now lots to do.

Our electric iron, oilskins and wellies are taken back to *Kalivala*, which is checked over, bidden a sad farewell, hoping she will winter kindly. We return to an invitation to Carl and Bella's apartment for dinner, together with some staff and their wives, as a combined house-warming and Christmas celebration.

I shake the creases out of my only dress and Sam's blazer and we scrub up well, to find on arrival, (not surprisingly!) that plans have changed. Bella is not now cooking the dinner, and Carl is not yet home. Hardly have we all introduced ourselves, taken a sip wine and nibbled an olive, when the voice on the intercom from the downstairs foyer loudly proclaims, "I am hungry NOW! We eat!" Carl is not a man you purposely displease, so with one accord the party downs its wine in one slug and we drive to Cassis to a renowned restaurant.

Even inside it is cold, the fillet steaks do not melt in the mouth, service is hap-hazard and Carl's barometer becomes set at stormy, thus the evening is rather an anti climax!

December 11th

In between washing, cleaning and packing, there is time for a last walk to Renecros bay to read and soak up the warm winter sunshine. I would have preferred to paint, but there is nothing sufficiently inspiring.

Our last evening is more convivial. We are taken, together with other colleagues to the familiar back street bistro, *Au Fin Gourmet*, which is warm and friendly, lives up to its name, and even Carl is in high spirits. We bid goodbye, wishing a happy Christmas to all, including the proprietress, who again declares her love for Sam.

December 12th

Early this morning Sam is to be found down in the bilges enjoying a last pump out session, whilst I fold and stow the bedding, check all sinks, loos and galley floor so as to avoid any adverse criticism.

The time comes to lock up *Hope II*, so with just one backward glance, we wipe out our footprints on the deck as we leave to be taken to the airport. The drive is uneventful except for the unnerving sight of a battered car, driven by an aged French peasant who is completely oblivious that he is speeding towards us in the fast lane of the motorway. And he waves!

The flight is on time, and by 5pm we are enjoying a proper cup of tea and reflecting on the last month. Has it been a complete waste of time or do you just make the most of any opportunity that presents itself?

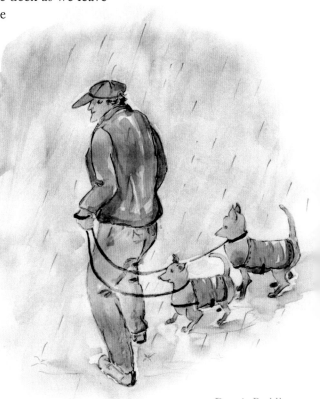

Doggie Paddle

Chapter 10
Autumn Fruits

August 8th 1993

Because we had paid for one year, we do not return in the spring as usual, and it is already august before taking the ferry from Portsmouth to Ouistreham. A hire car is waiting as an alternative to having the palaver of moving our own car every few miles. The heavy luggage contains English tea, instant coffee, salad cream, Marmite and two litres of anti-foul paint.

Being slightly late docking, we are anxious to make up lost time on the dual carriage way. About twenty miles along the road, a gendarme jumps out from an obscure gateway frantically waving his arms and blowing a whistle, and narrowly misses squashed toes as Sam comes to a grinding halt in front of him. "You were speeding," I mutter. "Not me, there must be an accident somewhere," Sam replies.

A peaked cap pokes through the window and after a polite *Bonjour monsieur*, words like *plus vitesse* and a translation of eighty kilometres speed limit, NOT one hundred and ten, filters through. Sam is marched off under escort to somewhere behind a farm house while I sit and wait. The gendarme re-appears, asks for my driving licence and suggests that I drive into the next town to the bank for the 600 franc fine,(about £60). "No way sir!" Reluctantly, I pull out this amount from the 1,000 francs we had just cashed on the ferry that I was hoping might last at least a week. I then have to go with him to the radar van sneakily hidden round a corner, to wait for the triplicated and stamped forms to be filled in by a callow cadet who is much harassed by our *Franglais*.

From then on, we take heed of every speed sign, with not so much as a, "Told you so!"

Signs for *Gites* and *Chambres d'Hôte* send us down pot-holed lanes with no visible habitation. A small hotel offers a room on the third floor, which is declined. All we want is a comfortable farmhouse with a homely, smiling farmer's wife. We are now weary, and suggest that at the next sign pointing to accommodation, we shall stop regardless.

This sign diverts us two and a half miles down a valley before drawing into a farm yard to scatter the hens and here, at last, is the imagined lady on the doorstep with her apron on, having just taken three king-sized quiches out of her primitive coal fired oven. This looks promising - or does it?

'Reception' is her husband in an off-white vest and baggy trousers, our room has just been 'modernised' - by lining it with pine boarding, and is quite attractive, but there are no signs of any other guests.

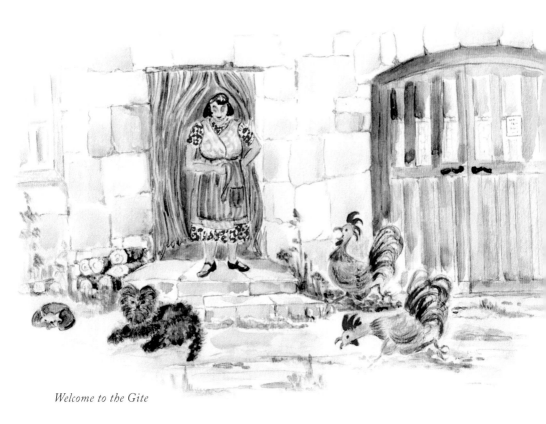

Welcome to the Gite

Dinner is not served until 8.30pm, so perhaps we could have a drink first. In the dining room, all the chairs are stacked up on a long bare table, so we go outside. The terrace is a small wrought iron table in the corner of the yard, where the patron, still in his vest, serves our drinks whilst the dishevelled dog sleeps by our feet and the fine, arrogant cockerels scratch round us. We try not to laugh too loudly.

At 8.30pm, the scene has changed completely. The lights are on, the long table is prettily set and *Papa* is wearing a crisp white shirt and smart black trousers as he hands out the wine lists. Twenty-eight people sit down to dine, *Mama* and *Papa* run from the adjoining kitchen with the various dishes. First come the portions of quiche, followed by vegetable pancakes, and mushroom omelettes - all freshly made - then there are numerous country cheeses, breads and the typical flan, all washed down with pitchers of a heady local brew. It is a strange gastronomic experience, and no one can say they are still hungry – podged, yes.

Soon everyone is chatting and laughing together, it is like a big party in spite of the different languages. We never saw them again; I think they came from the village.

The grand sum of £36 is painstakingly totted up after a breakfast of hot chocolate, croissants and home made jams served by the beaming wife.

The last leg of the journey back is taken via Valence in order to assess the marina for the possibility of wintering *Kalivala* next year, when we hope to start taking her up the River Rhone.

On arriving back to the boatyard at St Mandrier in the early evening, it is a shock to find that the hatch had been forced open and some tools are missing, and even worse, the gin, whiskey and beer bottles are empty next to two mugs containing cigarette ends. Some one has had quite a party!

At the *Capitanerie* they are very sympathetic and blame it on to the nearby military. Who knows? Once again we have been robbed, and it leaves an uncomfortable feeling.

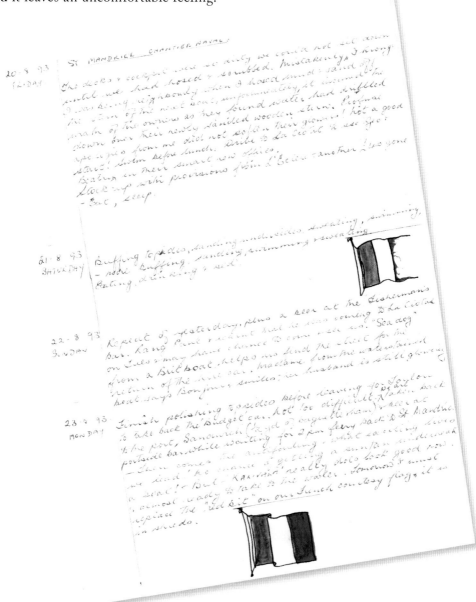

Sanding undersides, buffing topsides, sweating, swimming, more buffing and sanding before renewing the anti-foul, a messy task being akin to painting with treacle. *Kali* looks really smart now and ready to go back into the water, but I must remember to repair the shredded red end on the French courtesy flag.

Miming the stolen tools to Maurice on the next boat, provokes laughter on the pontoon and I hear words about *Les fous Anglaise*. Yes, I know we are fools.

A list is made to take to the Gendarmerie - we know the routine well by now, but we are not pleased to learn that there is no one in St Mandrier sufficiently high ranked to deal with it. (Perhaps they have no typewriter.) We are told to go to the Commisariat in La Seyne a few miles way, but having returned the hired car, it all proves too complicated, so we just post the insurance claim instead.

Every time we think about leaving, the weather turns against us and we are teased for our *mañana, peutêtre* attitude, perhaps we are becoming even more timorous in our dotage, or is it that time is not now of any great importance?

Days pass enjoying the company and friendship of the many assorted yotties on this pontoon, especially a somewhat bohemian couple of London east enders with a colourful and rather coarse sense of humour. They live aboard permanently on their old, cosy boat and become called the *Sea Dogs*.

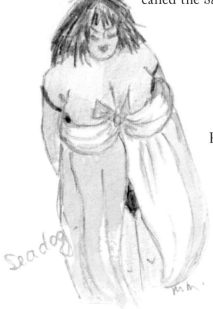

Seadog

For a touch of culture one evening, there is L' Orchestre de Chambre de la Philharmonique Slovaque de Bratislava performing in the little church. Sam reckons that it would be wasted on him, so I endure three hours on a very hard pew watching the intense expressions of six enthusiastic young men as they fiddle their way through *The Four Seasons*.

September 1st St Mandrier to Embiez

Today we say adieu to the *Sea Dogs* and others as we cast off for a return to Isle des Embiez following a naval destroyer leaving Toulon, which takes our wind from the sails. Once out from the sheltered inlet, there is a stiff headwind and tacking becomes tedious, so the motor goes on for the rest of the fifteen mile passage to the spacious marina.

A more thorough look at the island is taken with less effort by joining the rest of the tourists on *Le Petit Train* which trundles through pine woods, vineyards and rugged scrubland, passing small secluded coves and a set of man made ponds for marine biology research.

The peaceful atmosphere of this charming island lures us to stay for just another day, but the mooring fees and the prices of the poor quality fruit and vegetables is so inflated that to stay longer is not economic – especially with tonic water at £2 per bottle.

September 3rd Embiez to Sanary

In a strong breeze with sizeable waves, we head out into a beam sea but, since it is only a short distance across to Sanary, we tolerate the pitch and roll and just hold on tightly. On the helm, in spite of being able to see where we are heading, in jest I ask for a course to steer, which should not have been ignored, as somehow, navigation suffers a severe case of disorientation when Sam spots some masts in a marina and blames the compass. There follows a slight controversy but I obey my skipper, as one should, and helm over to enter this small port believed to be Sanary, yet it does not appear to fit the description. Finding no space and running out of depth, I do an about turn, churn up the sand and come out again into the rough sea. "Oh, well. We shall just have to motor on up to Bandol, it's only three more miles."

By now we are getting frequent 'wet ones' over the side, and the bottles and pans are rattling about below as we slowly make the approach to Bandol'. "Where is the aqueduct? Where is the Ile de Bendor?" We do not recognise anything, but at least it is a better harbour! Could this be Sanary, if so, where have we been?

We remind ourselves not to become too blasé about short passages, however simple they seem as eyeballs are not always as reliable as real navigation.

The impish wind thwarts all chances of a perfect manoeuvre stern-to into the berth, causing the man in the adjacent power boat to come scurrying out with an outsize balloon fender, and his girl leaps aboard to help fend off.

Once settled, we stroll into this slightly touristy but pleasant little resort with a good supermarket, excellent outdoor market and attractive squares. By the church door, Peruvian pan pipes trill in opposition to *Tannhauser*, The *Blue Danube* and *William Tell* gurgling from the organ on the ornate, gilded carousel in the shady square.

Further along, a lone guitarist strolls expectantly between the tables at the creperie. Music and the mixed aromas of herbs, roasting chickens, pizza, coconut, and fish, float from each bar and restaurant along the waterfront. The liveliness is enjoyable!

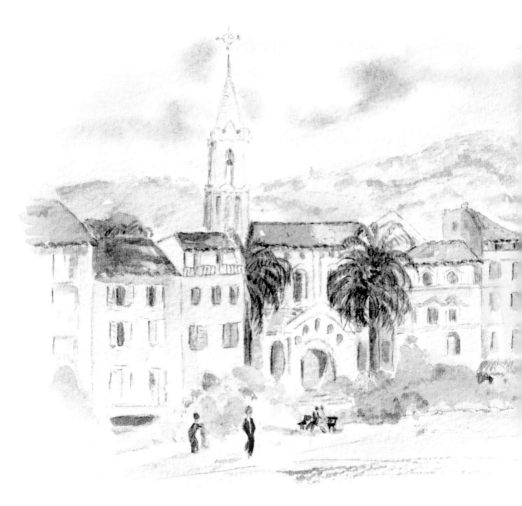

Sanary

September 4th

The surly *Capitaine* tells us that the weather is good for us today, so why do we stay. I give him my sad look and he reluctantly grants another night here.

The next day begins bright, so it seems a good time to sail a few more miles along, but by the time I return from the market, the breeze has stirred into a force five wind so we wait until afternoon and now waves are breaking in the harbour. The sky looks weird – we are not going any where in this! The *Capitaine* seems to be expecting us, and with a wagging finger he admonishes, "I told you it was a nice day yesterday."

Since it is not a beach day, we walk over to Six Fours, where chairs are all being set out for, "Oh, look. Another circus." In the car park, two llamas and a pony are tethered, ranging to and fro in boredom, and in cages nearby is a motley of fauna, i.e. two bad-tempered baboons, a mangy racoon, a scrawny scratching fox and a porcupine that has not enough space to turn round. The small boy being coached to do back flips and handstands does not appear to be full of enthusiasm. The scene has all the ingredients of the typical French family travelling circus, but we shall not be walking back here again at eight o'clock tonight.

The sun disappears and black clouds loom, bringing a momentous thunderstorm with torrential rain and through it, just discernible, is the tinny circus music; we are wondering what kind of tricks would a porcupine do? The storm lasts for three hours, so, perhaps the animals had a night off!

Due to persistent high winds, our stay here extends to seven days, and although Sanary is very agreeable, it is becoming a slight embarrassment to visit the volatile little *Capitaine* each day to admit that there is too much wind for us. With time he mellows, smiles and is almost friendly, then he brings us a gift – twenty four dustbin bags! How long does he think we are staying?

When the sea is too rough for swimming, one of our idle pastimes is to sit in the shady square watching the expressions and reactions of the children riding on the ornate carousel. At one time it had a steam organ, but now it is mechanical and plays havoc with Wagner. With the choice of galloping horses, elephants and Cinderella coaches, it is constantly busy, but the children's favourite always seems to be Leo the Lion with its immodest behind.

A *très chic* mademoiselle comes teetering along on her four inch heeled, white, open toed sandals. Head in the air, she tosses back her long blonde locks, daintily holding her designer handbag in her delicate fingers. *Quel domage!* With her nose so high in the air, she does not see the freshly turned coil of doggo lying in wait until too late, and she skids through the heart of it. "OOH – la – la – la laaaah, is the very Gallic verbal reaction to her dilemma as the malodorous mess of excrement oozes between her manicured toes!

Never before have we heard those words used other than in a French farce or cartoon, and certainly never with such depth of feeling! We do have a little sympathy as she limps away with remarkable dignity. I do not think that this needs a drawing!

The strong winds continue, the *Capitaine* now beams and winks at us when we pay for yet another night here, but if a three-masted schooner feels the need to shelter in the bay, then perhaps we are right to stay. An old power boat blows in and attempts to moor nearby, but the slender, nay, skinny lady on the bow does not seem to know what to do with her warps, which now looks like a pile of tangled knitting. They do not realise that they have to first pick up a chain, so they swing sideways and she is subjected to severe barking from her husband as we try to fend them off. This brings the *Capitaine* dashing down shouting angrily. The man shouts back, there is a shaking of fists and insults are hurled. We hear the word *chien* a few times, and there is an intense ding dong before they are safely secured. Whilst sharing this amusing diversion with another crew, a small catamaran deftly squeezes in beside us with two young men aboard, having just sailed down from Marseilles with all their kit on the trampoline, and are on the way to Nice. Here we are with thirty three feet of solid boat and won't sail eight miles down the coast because it is too windy – well, it does blow the crisps out of the bowl in the cockpit. Supper has to be eaten below, which helps to deaden the sound of the bongo drums!

We really must make an effort to move on tomorrow.

Circus tricks and Leo the lion
on the carousel

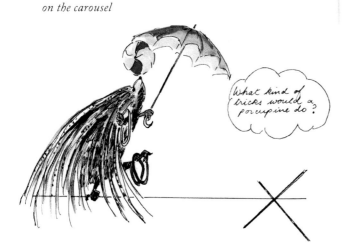

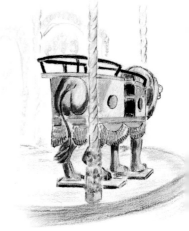

September 11ᵗʰ Sanary to St Cyr Les Lecques

September 11th Sanary to St Cyr Les Lecques

The day looks promising with just a few clouds and a light breeze but the fishermen say, "Mistral comes." Sam listens to the radio *Meteo* while I run round to the *Capitaine* to ask what his forecast says. (You would think we were crossing the channel not moving a few miles up the coast!) Now quite friendly, he predicts, "*bon* this morning, *un peu agite*, and *beaucoup* wind later." So Sam hesitatingly agrees to test it and we leave at 9. 20am. Apart from the force four headwind, and having to tack several times in an uneven swell, the hour and a half passage is stressless along this lovely stretch of coastline.

The wind funnels straight in through the narrow marina entrance. Reception is like a large plastic floating drum, and more than one minor obstacle is bumped before being able to grab it. The *Capitaine* can't help but notice our arrival and is quickly along to direct us to a berth and help to pull us into place.

Inspection of St Cyr les Lecques presents a pleasant little resort with a good surfing beach and the cleanest harbour we have seen yet, but then it does cost twice as much! The actual town of St Cyr is a three mile cycle ride away, and on this Sunday morning there is an extensive market selling everything but a good lettuce.

Further on, passing the ruins of a Roman villa we come to the small community of Madrague, which seems to be a cul-de-sac backed by mountains, up which we did not care to pedal, so make our return to the beach where the sea is warm and crystal clear for swimming. An English family, who we met yesterday give us a newspaper to catch up with events at home – who cares that it is three days old as long as they haven't done the crossword puzzles!

The forecast for tomorrow is *mauvais temps* – not good, and already the wind is piping up, tuning and orchestrating all the halyards, fenders, springs and reflectors to their own music as the black clouds roll in. The wind is not too fierce but one look at the narrow harbour entrance shows that it will be very tricky to pass through between those huge rollers beating against both sides. The *Capitaine* is expecting us when we go to pay for another night. It might not be a good day to sail, but wow, there is some magnificent surf roaring in, and we can't wait to get in it.

September 14th Les Lecques to La Ciotat

September 14th Les Lecques to La Ciotat

Looking over the harbour wall the sea looks tolerable. Since *Kalivala* needs a force four to get her going at full throttle, we burst through the heavy swell between the white water breaking on the rocky sides of the tight exit into a greater swell that proves quite bearable for the meagre three and a half miles.

To re-acquaint ourselves with this town, we walk through the main pedestrian street and see again the large leafed cauliflowers, the escaping snails and bubbling Paellas. The weeds are even taller round the derelict shipyard, which used to be the heartbeat of the town, the *pissoir* smells just as bad, and the Roman washhouse has been visited by many dogs. The park beyond is much improved, and we halt awhile to try and locate the cicadas which are noisily 'sawing off their back legs' in chorus up in the trees. They are difficult to spot, but look like out sized houseflies.

September 16th La Ciotat to Cassis

Leaving at 11.30am in a calm sea, all is serene until we reach beyond Ile Verte where a disturbed mess of waves and a headwind hits as we round the other side. Sails are reduced to jib only and the motor switched on. The entrance to Cassis is even narrower than Les Lecques. Surfing in on the crest of a wave with the sea breaking on rocks close to each side is quite a dry-mouthed experience.

All harbour staff seem to be at lunch when we tie up on the fuel quay, and we have to wait over an hour before filling up with diesel and being shown the only berth available. This is to lie across the end of the first pontoon inside the harbour where the boats are buffeting crazily. "Thanks but, no thank you," we tell him, so I run round to the other side of the inlet which is independently operated. Here we are offered two nights maximum, hanging off the end of another leg of pontoon, but at least the boats are not so restless, so we move.

The problem now is that our son, Paul who also works with Carl's company, is coming in five days time and wishes to stay on the boat with us. The *Capitaine* needs to see the ship's papers, so whilst in his office I put on a sad, pathetic face as I relate the situation, and gradually he wilts and offers to try and find spaces – and we need not pay until we leave! Having sorted him out, we reappraise the town, as it is now over three years since we were last here.

Crème de Cassis

Very little has changed, except that there is now more entertainment on the harbour side. Although quite common everywhere now it is the first time we have seen the live statues. A girl clad in off-white drapes with whitened face, arms and feet, stands motionless on a pedestal and moves only when money is dropped into her hopeful dish. She lets a faint smile slip when two elderly, disbelieving ladies dare each other to touch her foot. This creates curiosity in a very small boy, who then attempts to do the same, but the 'statue' bends down to pat his head, which frightens him and he runs off screaming for *Maman*!

After supper, a group of musicians are serenading the clients in a nearby restaurant with a big French horn, bassoons, cornets, trombones, tabor and noticeably more fervour than accomplishment. They oompah their way through waltzes, tangos and marches for over two hours, bringing the diners spontaneously to their feet to dance along the promenade to the very erratic tempo! Great entertainment until we wish to sleep.

Next day there is a different *Capitaine* on duty. He is young, with a pony tail, twinkly eyes and speaks good English. "Stay as long as you like," he smiles! It happens that we stay for almost three more weeks enjoying all that Cassis has to offer, and with much socialising.

Our son's visit is a short, happy interlude. He brings letters from friends and family, satisfies himself that he approves of the wine we buy, then takes us out for supper.

By the time we have been out for meals with Carl and other members of his staff for three consecutive days, and then reciprocated, we are ready to take a break from catering, which is just as well, since the refrigerator is having another fit of pique along with the shower pump.

Both are duly dismantled, prodded and coaxed, but the fridge does not succumb, leaving the Camembert cheese to permeate its pong throughout the boat, yet the chicken, which has been marinating in herbs, garlic and some three day old undrinkable wine is really good - although Salmonella did cross my mind.

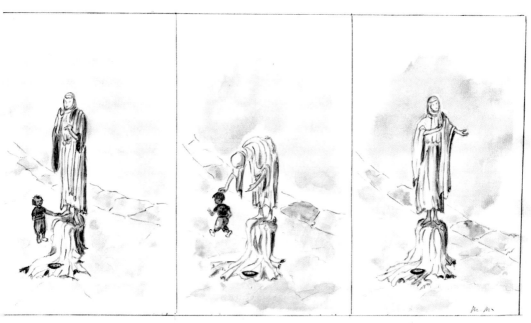

Living statue, Cassis

September 22nd

Storms are forecast. The rain begins in the early morning, when two charter boats arrive with at least nine wet crew on each, and only one chap seems to have the vaguest idea of what to do. No fenders are out, no warps ready so as is typical it is bump, "Allo. We are 'ere," and we have to help raft them alongside. Then they all need to go ashore several times and galumph, albeit courteously, across our decks each time.

Thunderstorms continue well into the night, and next morning when I go for the bread there is chaos in town. The streets are covered in sand, gravel and mud that has been washed down from the hills with the heavy rain, and the council are busy with large hoses trying to clear it, causing a traffic jam and there is much hooting and shouting.

It rains again onto our lunch, and again in the afternoon when a sudden deluge turns the downhill streets into rivers with waterfalls cascading onto the pontoon. Then the eighteen dripping yotties troop back across our decks full of mirth and wine.

September 25th

It is Sam's birthday today, he has three cards waiting at Poste Restante. I thought of treating him to some new shoelaces, but the mood faded in favour of some culture at the small museum. There is not a lot to see there but they do try very hard to make the few Roman relics dredged up from the sea, two Provencial life sized figures and a collection of local Santon dolls look interesting.

On the seafront, for the autumn rally is a procession of thirty, beautifully maintained 1930's *Hodkiss* vintage cars, and while we sit admiring them, another so called famous character of Cassis arrives. This is the 'Cat Man' on a Heath Robinson contraption that perhaps was once a bicycle. Its origin is now obscured by add on boxes, cages, ladders and hoops. Cat Man stops in front of a restaurant and for a good five minutes loudly vents a spiel about the *très dangereuse* tricks about to be performed by the four cats huddled in the two tiny cages.

One at a time, the cats sulkily deign to walk across a ladder and jump, nay, carefully step through a hoop, all of which takes only less than a minute. After a feeble ripple of applause, he passes his hat round, moves a few yards along to the next eatery and begins his eulogy again. I am not sure whether the clients of these four in a row restaurants appreciate the intrusion into their lunch with these *marveilleuse* skills, but he is now droned out by the exhausts and revving of the group of pony tailed and fringed motorcyclists who parade slowly past, posing on their gleaming *Harley Davidsons*.

Further down the quay, the La Ciotat lifeboat comes in and is inspected by a group of dignitaries carrying banners and dressed in their best green acrylic suits. They are joined by two stiffly uniformed, De Gaulle look-alikes who have been laying wreaths at the War Memorial. There is a painting exhibition in the town hall, a leather craft market in the square, where a coach is disgorging a crowd of English tourists who are wondering what to do, and today's living statue is standing motionless in his death-like drapes, being ignored by the passers by! There seems no need to seek entertainment to celebrate a birthday as it is all happening right before us, although we do light a candle later, just as a gesture.

The late sun on the steep cliffs and pine trees helps to make you understand why Cézanne and Van Gogh loved Provence, as the clear light is beautiful.

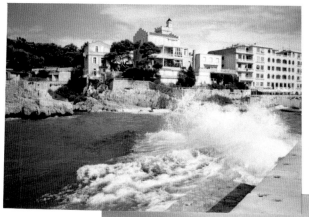

This page and next: Harbour entrance, Cassis

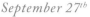

September 27ᵗʰ

Between storms, we enjoy walks over to the picturesque Calanques, which are deep inlets with a beach, crystal clear water and are backed by sheer steep cliffs, and during storms the waves cream over the top of the lighthouse and rocks making all the boats range around.

We have been thinking that it is time that we should be on our way to St Louis to get into the River Rhone before winter, but we hear that the rains have turned the river into a raging torrent, bringing down whole trees and much debris with it. Boats are not being allowed through the lock at its entrance from the sea. Perhaps it is providential that we are still in Cassis and should give up the idea of setting off up through inland waterways for this year. The problem however, with this harbour is that it is not well enough sheltered to leave a boat unattended for any length of time.

Reluctantly we realise that La Ciotat, yet again is the best option, that is if they will give us a berth for the coming winter. What a palaver! It is the ruling that the *Capitaine* has no say in the matter, and that long term berthing has to be sanctioned by the Mayor. After some hesitation we tell Carl of the situation. Luckily, because he has a business in the town, he is able to negotiate this for us and in a few days we hear that a berth has been allocated to us. Meanwhile, we can make the most of Cassis and its happenings.

September 29ᵗʰ

Weather conditions are perfect for sailing today, but we have been invited out to dinner by Carl and Bella, and we do prefer the atmosphere here. People-watching never ceases to astound, especially the ones with dogs.

The next day, "I told you we should have left yesterday!" The boats are all pulling and snatching as the south easterly swell lumps into the harbour, making the halyards tinkle. Twenty small schoolchildren wearing yellow oilskins, sou'westers and wellingtons troop down the quay for their dinghy sailing lesson, only to be turned away by their instructor, *"Pas aujour d'hui, mes enfants!"* (Not today my children.)

Two charter boats bump in for shelter with

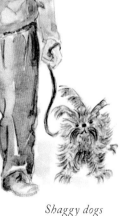

Shaggy dogs

207

much ado and lack of organisation, followed by a fishing boat, which has just collected in all the little yellow buoys that mark the swimming areas. Is this the sign that the end of another season has flown by? Well, we do need a blanket tonight.

Scottie dog

October 3rd Cassis to La Ciotat

Philipe, the jolly *Capitaine* asks if we are going now as the day is blue and beautiful, that is, inside the harbour. We still can't decide, there is a force seven wind blowing out at sea. The *Capitaine* tells us that he is about to take a 46ft yacht, single handed down to Hyères and here are we, dithering about a two hour passage down the coast. Whilst listening to the wind during the restless night, we conclude that we must be completely lacking in bottle!

Lucky dog

The day following, trying to prove to ourselves that we still have some zest left, we cast off the warps, drop the chain and leave through the almost back to normal, narrow channel. So far the wind is light, but the heavy swell rebounds off the high cliffs, causing a messy wave pattern. When the afternoon breezes stir,we are running downwind with a jib sail only, and our Loran instrument shows that we are surfing down the waves reaching an exhilarating speed of between eight and ten knots when passing between Ile Verte and Bec de l'Aigle. Just as we are enjoying it, all too soon we are in La Ciotat old harbour in just over one hour, clocking six and a half miles instead of eight, which is quite record breaking for the solid *Kalivala*. Sitting in the cockpit, we see two kingfishers fly by but more interesting, just a few feet away, is a van with a man shovelling out rat poison into the crevices in the rocks, and very apt, the name on the side of the van is *De–ratification*. This rat mobile continues to work its way through town and later, the pigeons are seen to be enjoying a treat.

Being the first boat inside, the south east wind brings the waves in, giving a most uncomfortable roll, and since we have not yet been given a permanent berth, we go over to the office to enquire. Our new berth, number 14 happens to be in the other, newer harbour, necessitating a very rough passage of at least four hundred metres to a much quieter position, but now the waves are breaking right over the wall, drenching us with spray – and the fridge motor needs prodding again. Ah well, you can't have everything.

Carl comes down to see us, (please don't ask Sam to go to the office) and his plan A is for us all to sail to tomorrow to St Tropez in *Hope II* for this year's Nioulargue, the races for large vintage yachts. Since the forecast is not good plan B is that we go by car and stay in a hotel overnight. Make a change we thought, whilst packing an over night bag.

At 8.30am we are ready and waiting, and waiting. At 10am we ring him and learn that he has now decided on plan C, and it is now to be on Friday.

On Friday, he is onto plan D, which is "tomorrow by car." Under my breath I said bad words pertaining to his parentage!

Returning from a brief dash to the supermarket in the rain, I return to be greeted by Sam and another man who I did not recognise until I had kissed him. It is Pierre who was going to be on the Atlantic shambles with us. He speaks no English and very fast French, but we think he says, "My place for drinks, 6.30pm. Pick you up."

He did pick us up and first we get a tour of the house, which is an interesting project since he is meticulously re-building an old house, using all the old bricks, stone and beams. In the grounds are also two more cottages, so he should be well occupied for several years.

Drinks linger on until nearly nine o'clock. His wife Janine, is easier to understand but Pierre speaks faster by the glassful but, by the end of the evening he can almost remember three words of English. Unable to keep our eyes open any longer, we bid our Adieus after having had supper, three hours of holiday films, and another hour of *Rive Gauche* music. All very sociable, but nearly nine hours of concentration and wine addles the brain cells.

According to Pierre, 'If a Mistral lasts through the night, then it will blow for three days. If it again blows through the night, then it will last for six days. Likewise, another night – nine days. It never starts in the morning, and never rains with it. During what is left of tonight, the wind is still screaming through the rigging and it is pouring with rain. Does that blow away that theory? Sam is wishing he had not mixed his grape with his grain.

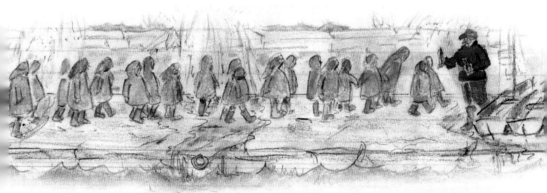

Pas aujour d'hui, mes enfants

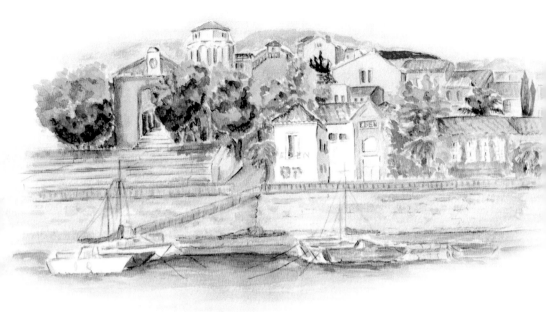

La Ciotat

Today is plan D day. The drive along the Corniche to St Tropez is very spectacular. Heather is in bloom, the leaves are turning to yellow, gold and red in the vineyards on the slopes, and there is snow on the mountain tops behind the town.

We are in good time to watch the spectacle of these two and three masted schooners, which are all the best classic yachts in the world, possibly up to two hundred in all. They vary in length from 100ft down to pretty little 15ft gaffers, and although we came last year, it is still a great sight to behold. Whilst watching the racing, it is difficult to know exactly what is happening when there are so yachts many milling about, and the appreciation is not the same from land as it is when you are on the water amongst them.

The atmosphere ashore is festive, a steel band plays *When the Saints*, the classic cars are there again, the usual row of *Harleys* are being admired, and a scruffy old man on a bicycle towing a pushchair, tries to play a guitar at the same time. It has been a pleasant diversion from rocking around on a mooring, even if it does start to rain again on the way back.

The wind pipes up and the six feral harbour cats on rat duty hide under the rocks. Perhaps it is some consolation to learn that England is also having much rain and flooding, at least it is warm here when the sun shines.

October 10th

Pierre brings a present for Sam, a second hand transformer that he has sought out from the Aladdin's cave of junk that will one day, become their bedroom. *Kalivala's* water heating system is such that, when motoring there is plenty of hot water, but when on shore power, the present unit, which was installed in America, takes a lower voltage so is not efficient. The excitement of a new toy sends us out to look for plugs, wire and switches. This needs a bit of miming when, at last, we locate a TV workshop within a dark doorway down a narrow cobbled street, which stocks all we need – second-hand for 25 pence. Soon it is ready for blast-off, and *voilà* – hot water. Sam tests it, and washes his feet with an ecstasy normally confined to the bedroom.

October 16th

Another end of season sign is that the newsagents have ceased to stock English papers, also one day can be hot and sunny and the next has a biting cold wind. The sea temperature drops to 58⁰ F, which sets us thinking that it might be time to start making arrangements to return home.

The adjacent boat owners, Rene and Claire, warn us that winter here can bring winds up to hurricane strength, and we should have some metal springs to lessen the force of the snatch on the mooring ropes. Rather reluctantly, we part with £25, but feel happier once they are fitted. Next, we pester the travel agent to find out methods and times for getting home, but come away with just too much confusing information.

An invitation from Rene and Claire for aperitifs proves very helpful, as they promise to keep an eye on our boat and keep the batteries charged up in return for bringing them a bottle of Cream Sherry when we come back next Spring. That sounds a fair deal! They also insist that we must borrow their car one day and have a day out.

The next few days are taken up with cleaning and sorting out the accumulation of duplicated 1990's magazines and leaflets from every information bureau from here to Capri. Train times and a date is eventually decided on, so we go to book it but the travel agent will not accept a credit card or a cheque. In the queue for the cash dispenser, we notice lots of people waiting and looking expectantly up the narrow street. What now? By way of advertising another *Merveilleuse Spectacle,* a large camel with floppy humps and bald patches, ambles its way drunkenly down making pedestrian progress frustratingly slow.

The girl taking our booking is attractive and most charming, but you can almost read her thoughts as we walk in with the cash, 'Oh sh**, not those English again.'

We invite Pierre and Janine for supper and fail to teach him a fourth word of English, but his hands speak volumes as he offers to store our bicycles for the winter. Having no holiday films to show them, we give them Pavarotte and Gilbert and Sullivan music instead. Then the wind comes, rocks the boat and spills the wine.

Sam eases off the warps, but just as we are settling down to sleep, he begins to worry about the bimini, as it feels as if we ready for lift off, and 1am sees us flapping about in night attire trying to take it off and tie it down!

It does not look an inviting day to go sight seeing but Rene and Claire, on the next berth, are becoming so insistent about taking their car that we leave for Castellet in the rain, but the Provence countryside is always a delight.

The vineyards in their autumn gold make patchworks of colour between the pines, Cyprus and olive trees against a backcloth of low mountains dotted with mellow pink houses and farms. Castellet is another small medieval, hilltop village which is famous for its old lavender distillery and has great charm. Every corner is a picture with pots of trailing geraniums and bougainvillea, old doorways, allies and archways that open on to surprise views across the valley far below. It, of course, also has a surfeit of gift shops, ateliers, artist's studios and all the other tourist trappings, but not at all brashly.

The racing car track, just a short distance away, is also owned by Paul Ricard. Lunch is a very filling Gallette, enjoyed in a small creperie with a cosy log fire in the corner.

Leaving the village, we think to take back an acceptable bottle of wine as a thank you gesture for the loan of the car. This entails bumping down two muddy lanes before finding the 16th century vineyard of Chateau Vanniere, where we have a sampling session in an old stone outhouse then, rashly buy three bottles.

On the way back is Cadiere, which is on the opposite hilltop, but it does not have the same appeal as Castellet. Taking the route via Madrague and Les Leques, we are back in good time to wash the mud off the car before the owners see it!

There is still time left to enjoy the daily way of life here. The eight year old schoolchildren come down most days for their sailing lessons in the harbour. With two or three to each dinghy, they are towed round in a circle and have to practice standing up, sitting down again, then rocking from side to side. There is much laughter and shouting, and always one who is over enthusiastic and falls overboard – usually a boy.

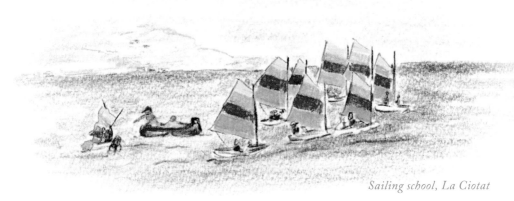

Sailing school, La Ciotat

Sunday morning is always a jolly scene, with queues at the butcher's and baker's, chickens being spit-roasted and metre wide pans of Paella bubble on a gas ring beside other spicy concoctions of stew. Everyone seems to be shopping for a feast as they carefully carry out their fancy boxes of gateaux, they make even more of an occasion with Sunday lunch than the English, and it all has to be fresh. Not so good is the dark red, half a tuna fish gazing with dead eyes at the flies on the catfish!

Sam extracts the ailing fridge yet again to take home for more repair; the sails removed, folded and stowed; anchors put down in their locker and the back of the cooker is dealt with – yuk! Pierre takes the bicycles to his home, nearly everything is packed and all that there is to worry about now is whether we can wake up at 6am tomorrow.

October 26th La Coitat to Hamble

All goes well, and when the train is running parallel to the River Rhone, we stand up in our seats to gaze in awe at the rate of the current and flooded fields. Whole trees are racing down in its turbulence, some of the marker poles have bushes stuck on the top,and masses of weed and debris are tangled in the shrubbery on the banks.

How thankful we are not to be in it as hoped. Perhaps we have made the right decision to leave *Kali* in La Ciotat after all.

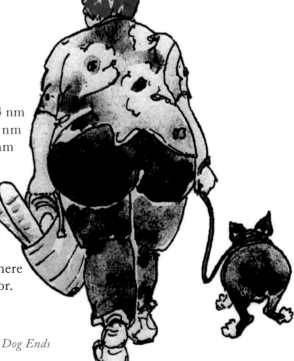

Statistics
6 times robbed
10 times visit the police station

St Mandrier to Iles des Embiez – 14 nm
Embiez to Sanary, plus detour – 5 nm
Sanary to St Cyr les Lecques – 8 nm
St Cyr to La Ciotat – 3.5 nm
La Ciotat to Cassis – 7 nm
Cassis to La Ciotat – 6.5 nm

Grand Total for 3 months = 44 nm

Not exactly record breaking, but there are a few day sails not accounted for.

Dog Ends

Chapter 11

Last course – Assorted trifles

Monday May 9th 1994

This time we bring the car again and after disembarking from the Duc de Normandy Ferry in Ouistreham, we drive down France through Argenton and Alencon towards Vendome, which looks interesting but we cannot see a hotel. In Blois we are weary with trailing up countless stairs at three unwelcoming, gloomy hostelries. Then we come across La Ville de la Tour on the side of the River Loire, which is owned by a charming young Italian who speaks perfect English. This building is 16th century with very low, old beams and death watch beetle, but it is clean and basic, what is more, Sam can see the car from the window! The town of Blois has a castle, attractive public gardens and interesting old streets of quaint timbered shops.

Driving on next day we pass through Amand, Montlucon, get lost in Clermont Ferrand and come to Puy, all is peaceful and pastoral with hedges of laburnum and fields of poppies. By the time we need to find a hotel, we have run out of scenery and into quarry land, then luckily see *Percedes* with a terrace looking out over the hills, just out of sight of the quarries.

On the third day of the journey, we make a stop in Viviers to look at the state of the River Rhone, and compared with the last time we saw it in October, the flow looked reassuringly gentle and peaceful.

At 3.30pm we are back on board in La Ciotat, and at first glance everything looks in order - but then we sense something. Surely I didn't leave coat hangers on the saloon seat, nor my water proof trousers on the chart table? Why is there a cigarette lighter on the floor when we don't smoke? As far as we can assess, the missing items are Sam's wetsuit, heavy waterproof coat, the hand held direction finder and my holdall. It is a most unsettling feeling to know that someone has rifled through your belongings! The *Capitaine* does not appear at all surprised; he thinks it happened in December and has an idea who the culprit might be but, having no proof, he can do nothing about it. It is not a very happy start to the season.

May 12th

Much work is to be done. The winter has coated the warps and fenders with oil and green algae, which now need to be scraped and scrubbed with bleach, then the sails are hanked back on and the bimini screwed in place.

Once more Sam replaces the repaired fridge motor, which at last seems to be working well. Noticing that the drinking water looks a bit like weak lager, we start to rinse out the tanks by standing on the seats, one each side of the cockpit, holding onto the shrouds, then get the boat rocking from side to side. The neighbouring boat people look pityingly at these crazy English, until we explain what we are doing, then they all agree that it is *un bon idee.*

With exposure to too much sun, the teak decking has become slightly warped in some small areas and needs replacing. The template is made out of a roll of very heavy, floral wallpaper bought from a most grateful lady in the market, and we wonder what the neighbours are thinking now.

Being worried about further break ins, the lock is strengthened and a devious device is set up involving a length of cord tied to a ring on the hatch inside the saloon then threaded through a drilled hole into the cockpit locker, which is then locked.

After re-splicing a frayed warp we are now ready to relax a while and attend any local happenings. The Ascension Day holiday weekend brings out crowds to watch the regatta, a spectacle of fifty old sail boats, including gaffers, schooners, and little lateen fishing craft with tan sails – who needs St Tropez?

In the square by the church there is another crowd, this is a jumble sale in aid of abandoned cats. Their 'antique' galvanised buckets at £25 each are not selling well. The proceeds from this special event go towards giving the feral harbour cats an occasional picnic in gratitude for keeping the rat population down.

The beaches are packed because of the sailboarding and kite flying competitions, which we stop to watch. It is all happening here today – except in the galley, where the fridge motor has died again.

On another business trip, son Paul has an overnight stay and takes us out for dinner, but the choice of restaurants here is somewhat limited. The surly maître d' brings the English menu, which is so comical that we have to ask for the French menu in order to translate it, for example: 'Two balls for your pleasure' gives you two scoops of ice cream with a choice of flavours. Other delicacies include, 'Pig salad' and 'Frolegs'. Our bursts of laughter bring about some raised eyebrows from the diners, and dour glances from the maître d'.

May 29th
Today is Mother's Day here, so after Sam has trimmed up the wobbly black sealant between the newly laid teak strips on the aft cabin top, we wander up to the park. A notice tells of a *Spectacle Speciale* in the open air theatre at 3pm, so we go along to see what it is, hoping that it is not another circus. At the gates I am presented with a pink rose, the same as all the other *meres* and *grand-meres*. The seats are on sloping ground under the shade of pine trees, and the stage is backed by a grassy bank and trees, all much nicer than expected. For more than two hours we are entertained by all the *Academies de Dance de La Ciotat*. The Ballet School is represented by twenty pretty girls flitting around the stage symbolising nymphs, Turkish delight and aphids. (Green fly and black fly?)

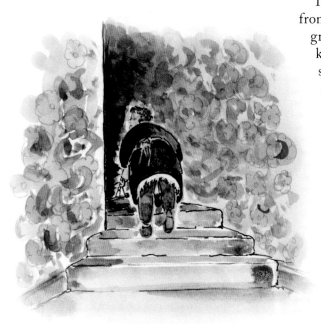

The classical music rasps out from a very worn, scratched gramophone record that doesn't know when to stop, and is just switched off suddenly with a crackle and a screech. Next comes Madame Pauline raunchily belting out a selection of Edith Piaff songs, and very good she is too. Following on, is some very physical disco dancing by a group of cheeky little movers all under ten years old. The afternoon has given an enjoyable taste of *la vie Francaise*, even if it was a bit corny!

Blois

Je voudrais regarder la chambre,
s'il
vous
plait

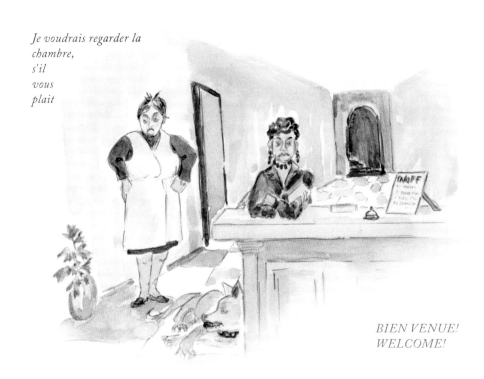

BIEN VENUE!
WELCOME!

June 10ᵗʰ

The wind blows hard all night, screaming through the rigging in furious lumps making it feel like living in a signal box on a mainline express railway.

Force 10 – 11 gusts are forecast, the semaphore on Bec d'Aigle is already experiencing a force 10, and two 40ft ketches are dragging anchor in the bay, yet it shows only a force 8 in the harbour.

It seems like a good day to drive over to Port St Louis to see what awaits us at the entrance to the River Rhone. It takes an hour to traverse Marseille due to trying to take a short cut. At Martigue, the Etang de Berre, which is usually a placid lake, is now a seething sea of white horses.

On arriving at Port St Louis we chat to an old caretaker, who advises on the best marina and gives us the address of a shipyard which is run by two English brothers. Finding them, they are extremely helpful giving advice on dis-masting and recommend that the best time to enter the Rhone is in mid August before the thunderstorms, yet after the snow has melted on the mountains. Looking at the marina right in the town, it is some consolation to find that it appears to be better than envisaged.

On the way back, we call in at some of the small ports that might be useful stopovers, and now feel more optimistic . A taxi driver's strike blocks the only route we know through Marseille on the way back – lost again!

June 13ᵗʰ

The weather is more settled now and the town is waking up for summer. The taps on the beach showers are turned back on, the newspapers are in stock and the harbour staff, in two boats, are towing out the yellow marker buoys and strings of corks for the swimmers, water ski bikers and small craft. One boat seems to be skippered by the bossy harbour dog who barks out orders, he is a scruffy mismatch between a poodle and a spaniel. We call him *Spoodle* – what else?

Our mail comes via Carl's office, or to the *Capitainerie* after being left for several days in the Mayor's parlour. We are waiting for Henri, the *Capitaine* to write a letter for us to send to our insurers asking for a claim form for the stolen items, and we are upset to learn that he wants us out of this port by July 1ˢᵗ. Now what do we do?

The well-practiced crocodile tears on his shoulder, an appealing gaze into his eyes and he melts, so before he changes his mind we pay for another month.

Taking advantage of fair breezes and calm seas, we have several short jollies out, sailing round Ile Verte, heaving to, and enjoying being afloat again as I had almost forgotten what to do first! Sam is becoming very adept at reversing into our marrow berth, but not yet with quite the speed and aplomb of the French sailors.

The sea temperature is now bearable for swimming, if you can thread a way through the well oiled shining flesh without offending anyone, to reach a space in the water with no bat and balls, or frisbies!

June 21st

All this week is supposed to be *La Ciotat Film Festival* - in competition with Cannes, no doubt!

Four films are to be shown in the crumbling Eden cinema, which is usually left derelict. We really should not scoff, as this is reputed to be where it all began with the Lumière brothers, inventors of cinematic photography, and they have a proud monument here. In this same cinema is an equally exciting Postage Stamp exhibition which takes up all of fifteen minutes, and coming soon is another Art Show – there is no shortage of entertainment!

One morning, chairs are being set out in the square for an orchestral concert, so at 11am we take our places sitting on the steps to listen to music from La Traviata, Madame Butterfly, The Merry Widow, and onto La Mer, and Yesterday. This is a relaxing and enjoyable selection, all played with much enthusiasm and slight lack of polish, as they get a bit lost on a few occasions!

June 23rd

A piece of cardboard strung to a tree says *Feux de St Jean 9.30pm in the church square*. We wonder what that is? Since it is only across the road, we go to sit on the church steps and wait. The origin of this event is obscure, but promptly at the given time, from down the hill come a band of fifes and drums, followed by a long procession of men, women and children all very colourful, in traditional Provence peasant dress. Two groups dance to rollicking tunes squeezed out from three accordions as they celebrate the lighting of the fire, thus sending flames, sparks and billowing smoke amongst the dancers from a huge pile of logs.

They are depicting the work of the seasons – sowing the seeds, hoeing, raking, thrashing, and spinning, followed by more charming dances from the different regions of Provence.

The fire burns enthusiastically, with sparks flying high, threateningly close to the hay, but no one appears concerned. Songs are sung, then the local children dance in a corner, to be later almost dragged off their feet by their exuberant elders. Amid dense clouds of smoke, the last dance is the *Farandole*, some of the audience join in - it rather resembles the Conga.

After more than two hours of thoroughly enjoying the regional customs, we suddenly become aware of the numbing effect of the stone steps on our behinds.

June 29th

In fond recognition of our 44th wedding anniversary, my bouquet of flowers is some lavender, filched from a handy flowerbed; it sits on the breakfast table in a beer bottle vase. It's the thought that counts.

Then we have visitors, Rene and Claire from the next boat. We feel that it needs explanation, as they already think that the English are weird. A short time later, they come back with a bottle of champagne, which presents the problem of – do we drink it now, share it or keep it for later? Being provident (or tight fisted) we will take it home for Christmas!

It is very hot; we drive up to Castellet in hopes of finding cooler air on the hill top and in the narrow shady streets, but soon become bored with all the garish paintings in the many art galleries, and it is just as hot up here.

Later, after a refreshing swim we are invited out for ice creams by the family on the other side of us, and that is all the excitement we have had on this special day.

July 8th

Despite prodding, poking and speaking roughly to it, the fridge motor again lies on the table in pieces and is finally pronounced dead, meaning that we must now submit to buying a new one. Pierre kindly offers to take us to a shop he knows in Marseille, where we take the plunge. I suppose it really is worth the three hours of rapid French earache just to be able to have firm butter and ice in a gin and tonic.

To escape the heat we occasionally drive up to the Route des Cretes, this is an area of paths on the top of cliffs 1,000ft high giving *Wow* views over to Cassis on one side, La Ciotat on the other and is almost level with the kestrels and swallows.

Terraces of small fir trees are carpeted with heather, rosemary, scabious, pinks and broom. Myriads of butterflies flutter by, the red admiral, peacock, brimstone and tortoiseshell butterflies are identified, but some blue, black, brown and grey ones we have not seen before. Giddyingly far down below, a few yachts are bucking on the white horses, and the only sound is the ceaseless chorus of the rasping cicadas.

Tonight, the open air theatre is performing the ballet *Coppelia*, we had intended to go but apathy prevailed. The music drifts across at dusk – a crackly recording which sounds very much like the original 78rpm gramophone record. Perhaps we have saved our kitty £12.

July 11th

Janine and Pierre come to supper, and mistakenly we introduce them to gin and tonic. *Très bon* they say as they knock it back like lemonade. Normally, Pierre speaks even faster after a glass of wine but tonight, the gin gets to him first and he falls asleep between courses. However, they do offer to store our car when we leave until we are able to fetch it.

At 3.30am I am abruptly woken by Sam kneeling on my calf and saying, "There is someone up on deck." He puts his head up out of the hatch and sees a man cutting off one of our best fenders. The Franglais conversation that follows now sounds comical, but at the time we are very afraid of what a man with a knife might do. "That is my balon," says Sam. "Is it *très importante* to you?" is the reply. "Yes. Put it down." "But I am a fisherman, I need it for my work!" "It is mine. I need it also for my boat," says Sam as he pokes a small length of aluminium tubing through the gap in the hatch, hoping it looks like a gun barrel. It obviously frightened him, as he just put it carefully down, leaps off, then casually strolls away.

A few minutes later, a security patrol van comes along and we relate the story which is received with the typical shrug. The large Alsatian dog lazing on the back seat, shows no enthusiasm for a chase either. Restless and a little frightened, we wonder if he did only come for a fender or is he the same thief who has taken our other things? The *Capitaine* is most apologetic, but of course, it is not his fault.

July 13th

There is a happening on the Place d' Anglais! Eight little rowing boats from Embiez have landed here and are being greeted by a band and the local majorettes. With more batons on the ground than in the air, they perform their routine to a repetitive tune that is reminiscent of the Church Lad's Brigade on the march. We should not laugh, but it is interesting to see how seriously it is taken – as is yet another art exhibition in the Chapel of the Blue Penitents across the road!

The next day is Bastille Day, a national holiday, so there is even more activity. There is a parade of *Le Ligue de droits des hommes*, which we think might be about the Rights of man. A flashing police car heads the same group of majorettes, still dropping their batons, and the band are playing the same tune. They are followed by sauntering sections of the armed forces, two flag bearers, the Mayor and Mayoress and a straggle of civilians. I'm sure it has an important significance that we do not fully understand. In the old port is a Craft Fair but as I do not need a plastic sundial, a Tutankhamen mask, plaster animals or weird jewellery, I did not open my purse.

Fireworks whizzed, popped and banged spasmodically well into the night, accompanied by the multi decibel pop group blasting out from a waterfront bar.

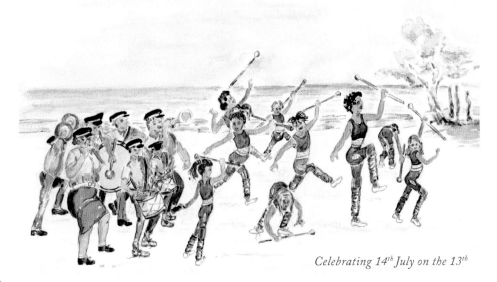

Celebrating 14th July on the 13th

July 16ᵗʰ

Many posters and leaflets all round town are proclaiming *Inauguration de Port de Pleasance at 11am* and since that is on our patch, we must attend!

This event happens to be the official opening, by the Mayor, of the new traffic barrier into the marina. It is well attended by a handful of curious onlookers, including ourselves, the harbour staff and *Spoodle* the dog. The mayor makes his speech, a cheer goes up as the fist car passes through, then he shakes hands all round and wishes us *"Bon vacance."* (Good holiday.) He cannot know that we have been here for weeks at his sanction.

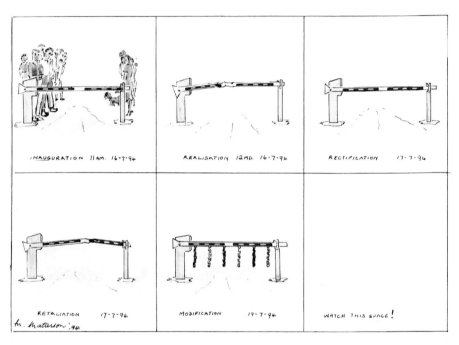

Installation of the barrier

There is time before lunch to browse round the market at the familiar scenes. Instead of budgerigars, there are collared doves having to stand three deep in a tiny cage, the tortoise has done a back flip off the table again, but the snails are not so frisky today. We could have wild boar for supper - he looks wild being cooped up in that small cage, the goat next to it does not look too pleased either, and the Peruvian Panpipes are exciting the ducks and hens to be all a flutter. It is really quite sad, I could not possibly buy meat while it is still alive, but they do here.

Further up, the advertised Music in the street is tuning up and first we come to the Organ grinder (no monkey!), who unwisely, is standing too near to a group of young flautists so you cannot hear who is playing what. A little way on are five violinists, then a saxophonist who are all members of a school orchestra on a course – they certainly need it.

On our return, it is obvious that already, an unobservant motorist has been unaware of the new barrier, as it now has a big bend in the middle.

It is so easy to become absorbed with the day-to-day events that we are forgetting to plan our departure. Mañana is the word! Each day we see the same people pass by and give them names.

Madonna of the rocks

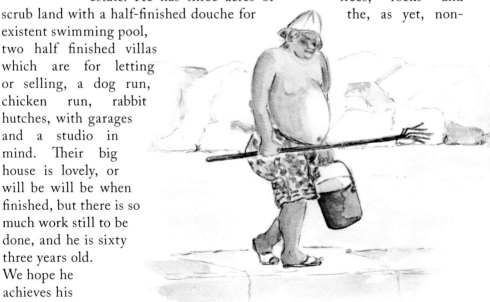

In particular there is the large lady who suns herself, Madonna of the rocks and the fisherman with the long fork is Neptune.

We cannot leave yet, we are still waiting for the letter for the insurance claim and then there is tomorrow's spectacle of the high wire act, the bungy jumping at the Place de l'Anglaise, Paul will be here again next week, and now Janine and Pierre have asked us to supper. There is just too much going on!

Pierre takes us round his grounds - almost an estate. He has three acres of trees, rocks and scrub land with a half-finished douche for the, as yet, non-existent swimming pool, two half finished villas which are for letting or selling, a dog run, chicken run, rabbit hutches, with garages and a studio in mind. Their big house is lovely, or will be will be when finished, but there is so much work still to be done, and he is sixty three years old. We hope he achieves his dream.

Neptune

July 20ᵗʰ

At last, Henri, the *Capitaine* comes along with the awaited letter, so we can now take the car to Pierre's and prepare to leave. On the way we make a detour via Les Cretes to take in the last views from the top and walk through the butterflies. Then the clouds roll in bringing a potent thunderstorm, which cancels the evening Marionette Theatre featuring Guignol, the French equivalent of Punch.

There is still time for a few more swims, where Sam surveys the beach scene with his usual comments of "Blimey! Cor! Wow! Disgusting!" and "Gordon Bennet!"

Another circus is being set up, we see the caged vans containing a pacing tiger, a family of monkeys preoccupied with a grooming session, a bare-arsed baboon and a large black bear ranging stressfully from side to side. Poor creatures, are they ever let out of their cages? I suppose that the lopsided camel and the haughty llama fare a little better by being tethered outside in their own personal pile of dung. We do not think we shall be attending this show tomorrow night.

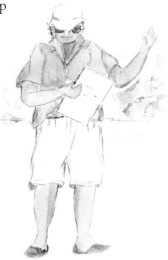

"Ici votre lettre"

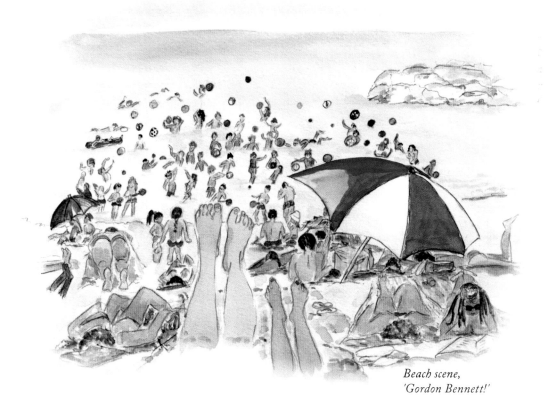

Beach scene,
'Gordon Bennett!'

Chapter 12

Leavings

August 1ˢᵗ

All psyched up to leave, we take Henri a bottle of whiskey and a drawing of
himself, with some chocolates for the two office girls and we say our Goodbyes,
only to be told, "Meteo not good. Do not go!" Such an anti climax – but, as
it happens he is right, and the waves are soon breaking over the rocks of the
harbour wall and frightening the cats. Madonna and Neptune do not pass by
today.

August 2ⁿᵈ La Ciotat to Ile de Frioule

On this bright, sunny morning it is with very mixed feelings that we drop the
chains, wave to our friends and leave the harbour. The *Capitainerie* staff are
still waving from their balcony when we reach the fairway buoy.

As expected, the pleasant, moderate wind is on the nose with just a slight
swell, so we let the motor do the work whilst crossing the picturesque bay
of Cassis instead of taking time to tack. After three hours, taking the inside
passages past Ile Jarre and Ile St Marie, we see an old signal station and
many grim gun emplacements, which are relics of the last war. Once round
the headland of Cap Croisette, the motor is cut to sail comfortably at five
knots with just the *Genoa* sail, in spite of the choppy sea breaking over the
foredecks.

When the marina on Ile de Frioule is a quarter mile away, we are taking in
the *Genoa* when the furling rope breaks, leaving the big sail flapping noisily
as I try to hold it down – engine on quickly to mill round and round while
Sam somehow, temporarily fixes it. Then we continue and tie up alongside a
concrete jetty in a concrete marina in what looks like a has-been quarry.

The *Capitaine* is plump and laid back, his only two English words are, "No
problem," and only charges £5, so the place looks better already! The stony
beach where we swim also resembles a disused quarry, but apart from the ferry
disgorging tourists from Marseille every half hour it is quite peaceful here.

The next morning is spent sorting out warps, to try to find one long enough
to repair and refit the furling gear, then scrubbing the salt off the decks from
yesterday's sail. Recovering our breath, we sit with a coffee in the cockpit
surveying the moonscape beyond the neat modern promenade, the one bar
and small shop. There must be more to Frioule than this.

Walking out of the marina, we pass by the sewage plant and a power plant
to climb a stony path between barren white rocks and are not overjoyed with
the place. "Just one more corner and that is enough." Surprise! Here, the

scene changes, there are lovely secluded anchorages and pretty inlets with clear turquoise water, where the compulsion to jump in to it becomes too irresistible, despite being unequipped. In ninety degrees of heat, it only takes a few minutes to drip dry.

Further on, we see the little tourist train and track the puff of blue smoke as it labours up the hill. Following its direction for over a mile, we wonder if there is anything interesting up there. Eventually we come to an old ruined building which is now being restored, it was once Hospital Caroline for tropical diseases. Across from the hospital, down a steep path is a secluded cove, Calanque d'Esteve, complete with diving raft, showers, a bar and lifeguards! So there is life on Frioule after all – we wondered where the ferry loads disappeared to!

August 4th Ile de Froiule to Sausset les Pins
There is just time to fetch a baguette before we cast off at 10am on a hot cloudless, calm day. We shall enjoy this!

Half a mile outside the harbour, the heating alarm bleeps once and is ignored, then it becomes more insistent on attention, and we realise that there is no water coming from the exhaust pipe. With the engine off, we flop around whilst Sam makes a brief check but is unable to find a cause. Slowly, slowly, we return to spend a very uncomfortable hour and a half with heads down in the engine compartment cleaning filters, and screwing and unscrewing nuts and bolts sited in the most impractical positions, and only one screw is dropped to eternity into the bilges. When the impeller has also been checked, we are ready to resume the passage.

By this time there is a nice breeze to give a leisurely sail, tacking a few times before reaching Carre le Rouet port in mid afternoon, only to be courteously turned away because it is full. Sausset les Pins is only a further two and a half miles, so we give up being purists and motor briskly before that marina also becomes too full.

What a nice surprise it is to be welcomed on entry, directed to a berth and helped to moor up, but it has taken almost all day to make fifteen miles of progress.

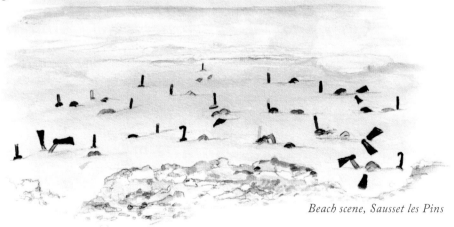

Beach scene, Sausset les Pins

This fishing town and resort appears to be mostly modern, non-descript yet dominated by a castle. The evening is filled with the sounds of house martins as they come in to roost in the *Capitanerie*, together with the bar singer who has much enthusiasm but very little voice.

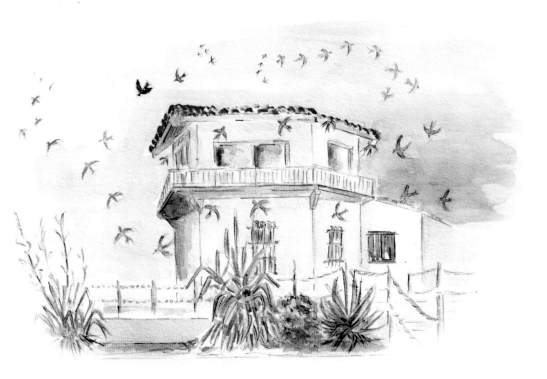

Twilight at Sausset les Pins

August 5ᵗʰ

If we cannot sail into Carry le Rouet then we will cycle there. It is fairly flat with a pleasant coastline, but we never reach the town as some daunting hills confront us at a confusing roundabout and we give up, it is too hot for hills.

Back in Sausset, we find a beach with showers, lifeguards and a bar, but it also has very weird, lumpy, moonscape rocks, making access to the water painfully difficult and relaxing barely possible.

It is a treat to have a new shower block and toilets handy to the boat, but it is so new that the notices depicting *Dames* and *Hommes* are not yet in place, so it is a bit confusing – but interesting.

"Oh, no! They have caught us up again." The circus is in town and it is happening right behind us. The children doing acrobats, the frightened goat balancing on an eight inch table, the haughty llama choosing its own circuit and the supercilious camel deigning to saunter reluctantly to and fro – haven't we seen these somewhere before?

Regardless of the clouds and waves breaking at the port entrance, we leave. It is a bit lumpy but for once, the wind is in a favourable direction from the east, then just as we are unfurling the jib, the warning sound from the cooling system bleeps again. We thought we had cured that problem! The attempt to sail back to Sausset drives us too near to the rocks, and it is now a headwind, so gently we motor back to set about the problem once more.

Sam spends the next four hours checking every possibility, then tries to remove the water pump without having the right sized spanner, and is lent every size but the right one, until a man from the boatyard kindly finds one. A bolt has to be sawn through and a slipping bush is found on the impeller that was not previously spotted.

With good directions, we find the chandlery for a replacement – out of stock – but we are promised that one will be here tomorrow.

It is quite a surprise at 8.30pm this evening, when a shout from the dockside is from the chandler, who has come down with our new impeller. Today we are thankful for the kind people, prompt service, and that we have hopefully cured the problem before coming to the River Rhone. The wind direction has changed also, making life more comfortable in the harbour.

August 9th Sausset les Pins to Port de Carro

An early rise. Sam fixes the new impeller and also removes a wad of weed from the thermostat. At 8.30am we are on the way and the pump seems to be working well. Outside the harbour, the light breeze becomes a fluky wind and the gentle swell grows into a big cross sea with two metre high waves, which throw us about unkindly.

From being a pretty coastline, the land now flattens out giving the impression of falling off the end of the world and making the hour spent sailing the last four miles seem like an eternity. Luckily, a boat is just vacating the only space on the jetty, and a jovial *Capitaine* takes our lines.

The small town resort looks attractive, except for the higher prices in the shops. This port is said to be sheltered, but the now very rough sea washes a canoeist up onto the rocks of the harbour wall and splashes over the top, encrusting our hair and boat with sticky salt water. Every boat is now bucking and snatching on their warps and it is spilling our drinks, so going for a walk is the better option.

To the west of town is a rocky beach backed by heathland and to the east, nearer to town, is a small sandy cove where crashing surf is being enjoyed by lots of laughing, screaming bodies as they tumble up the sand. We join them!

Chapter 13

Last Course

August 11ᵗʰ Sausset les Pins to Port St Louis

The morning looks fair, but another Mistral is forecast for the afternoon so, as it is only thirteen miles, perhaps we can sneak off before it starts. The wind up the stern gives an insidious rolling motion, not very pleasant but bearable.

For the first time we are having to keep a constant lookout for close encounters with oil tankers and cargo ships. The panorama has changed to sights of ugly masses of chimneys, power stations, oil refineries and storage tanks – a totally different world.

The direction finder whistles its alarm, "Shut up, we are trying to concentrate," but it is only trying to tell us that we are off-track in the midst of a confusion of buoyage to be identified. After some concern, the eastern lala buoy is located, which has a very obscure top mark, then the northerly one is clearly defined where we alter course for the St Louis lighthouse before turning into the stretch of canal. It is now that the water cooling alarm starts up again - after all the attention its had too. We slow down, unfurl the jib and amble slowly up the three miles of canal. Halfway up is the boatyard which we had previously seen, owned by the two English brothers, so we call in and arrange a day for taking down the masts ready for the river.

The marina in the town is adequate, with a helpful *Capitaine* who gives us a key to the toilets and showers, which are the coldest ever.

Tonight we have to fix up the netting to repel the voracious hordes of St Louis mosquitoes.

August 12ᵗʰ

Whilst I am tackling the laundry, Sam's morning play is to unclog more weed from the thermostat and then create an awful mess as he scrapes out the furred-up inside of the water jacket – surely that should cure it!

This rather strange town has developed around the St Louis tower, which was erected to defend the mouth of the Grand Rhone in the 18ᵗʰ century before the docks were built in 1863. To find a shop, we walk along, criss crossing disused railway lines on crumbling roads past a derelict warehouse and the Dockworkers' Union Club, where a few old men are playing boules on a small patch of gravel. A lonely, shaggy brown pony with flies in its eyes, grazes lazily in the adjacent small enclosure. This is certainly a much different scene to that we have become accustomed; they say the town is trying to restore itself – perhaps we have not yet walked far enough!

The tower is the main feature of the town and it also serves as the information bureau. We pay £1 to climb to the top where, looking with binoculars, we can see over the vast flat area of the Bouche de Rhone on one side, and mountains on the other. The calm canal runs to the sea like a bright blue ribbon with the river beyond and we try to estimate the speed of the current by timing the rate that the seagulls float down – two knots is a very rough estimate.

Returning, we find, with much apologising that our electricity supply has had to be forfeited to help feed banks of arc lamps and amplifiers for a pop concert on our quay. We have two hours of peace before the group and their thousands of decibels reverberate their bass thumps throughout the boat. The audience appreciate it, and it is really quite good, ending with a firework display at midnight.

August 14th
Our days are now busy making ready for a different way of life on the river. All available fenders are rummaged from the bottom of the locker and the sails are unhanked, folded and stowed. Reluctantly, we have to undo all the fancy rope work that we knotted round six feet of mast that comes down through the centre of the saloon table and into the floor, otherwise the mast will be too difficult to take out.

Two lengths of sail cloth are tied to the stanchions on each side to protect the fibreglass hull from being scuffed by the fenders when in the locks.

August 16th
This beautiful morning would be the perfect time to set off, but today is booked to have the masts taken down in the boatyard on the canal. To be able to make the supporting cross trees, chaps at the boatyard have to go out to fetch the wood, giving us time to exchange reading books in their office *library*, then read while waiting longer for them to be made. At midday they disappear for lunch then, at last, at 1.30pm the crane trundles in and we have hot, anxious gasps as the masts, in turn, dangle and swing precariously over the three fitted supports on the bow, stern and coach-roof, to be lowered into place. First, there is too much mast protruding over the stern, and now more than wanted over the bow, but we shall have to be careful. The shorter mizzen mast is lashed along the main deck. Job complete, they give us an updated weather report, which tells of a Mistral starting tomorrow and advise us to delay the departure as that is the wind that funnels straight down the Rhone. We pay £45 for their services, which is much less than expected.

As we pull into our berth, Neil, the *Capitaine* brings down three faxed letters, two from family and one from the insurance company which says the letter from Henri, the *Capitaine* at La Ciotat, does not fulfil their requirements, and they still require a letter from the police. "Drat!"

The day rounds off with a 'happy hour' spent in the company of two fellow countrymen on their way to Spain, followed by the whole of the Viennese

Night Concert from the Albert Hall, broadcast by the French radio – most enjoyable.

August 17th
The Mistral does not happen, we could have left this morning, but now we need to go to the police station again. Given directions lead us across the railway lines and past the boarded up warehouses into a street with a few trees in it – that is a pleasant change, but what a shame there is a sparrow, claws in the air, lying dead in the gutter. A few steps further along there are two more – poor things, there must be a hawk about.

Inside the *Gendarmerie*, we explain the situation in best school French, which takes a little time to dawn on the two uniforms at the desk. They have a discussion then direct us to the *Gendarmerie Nationale* office a few yards down the road, where we go through the whole story again, only to be sent upstairs to yet another office.

The door is open, revealing a middle aged upholder of the law sitting gazing out of an open window with a rifle resting across his thighs. He seems to be a little piqued at the interruption of his present occupation of shooting sparrows. Going through our story for the third time, he starts asking questions and we struggle to explain why it has taken so many months to report a robbery that took place fifty miles away. However, with one eye still looking out of the window and one hand on the rifle, he manages to type a plausible letter with one finger, then bids us a cheery "Adieu", and turns back to give the sparrows his full attention before we are even out of the room.

The letter is promptly posted, and we can again begin to psyche ourselves up for the morning departure.

August 18th
There is a queue waiting for the *Capitanerie* to open at 8am as everyone seems to be wanting a weather forecast. The crews sailing easterly go away happy. For us he gives, north-westerly wind force 6, which means straight down the river. "Do you have to go?" he asks. "Then don't!" Another anti climax.

Resigning ourselves to another night in this unlively resort, we walk along the riverside to look at its state. "Hmm, perhaps he is right!"

Returning by the fish boats, potholed roads, drab hotels and the old pony, we think we have now exhausted the attractions of Port St Louis, and our spirits are low.

The bright moment comes in the evening when the very kindly *Capitaine* visits to tell us that, 'his children can leave tomorrow. The meteo is good for you!'

And so it is on August 19th 1994 that we are milling round with dry mouths, waiting for the swing bridge to lift at 8.30am to pass into the lock. Never having been in a lock before, we had not expected the walls to be so high and were not as well prepared as we should have been. Our warps are too short, I cannot reach the bollards and it is all a bit embarrassing to have to be helped by a power boat crew!

This is it. We are now on the wide, tree-lined River Rhone with egrets and herons; we are ticking off the numbers on the kilometre marker posts along the twenty seven mile stretch up to Arles. At last we are on our way to take *Kalivala* home to Hamble with the refrigerator and engine working well. The rivers and canals present a totally different aspect and way of life as we are soon to discover – but that is another story!

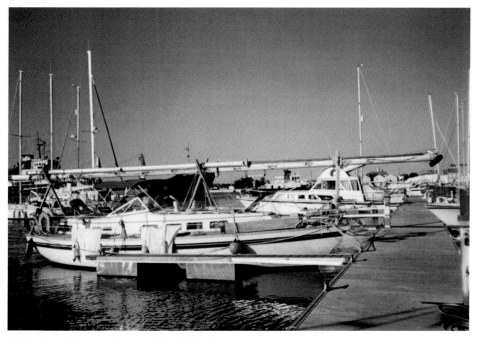

Kalivala with masts down at Port St Louis

P.S. When we reach Valence, Sam takes the train to La Ciotat to collect the car from Pierre, and we leave the boat in Valence for the winter and drive home.

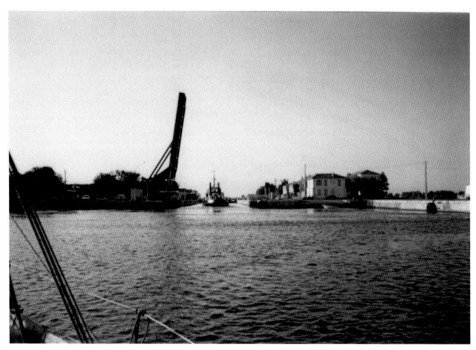

August 19th 1994
Lifting bridge and lock leaving St Louis

Footnote
If I have seemed to be a bit disparaging about some of the places and events, I apologise for any offence, but remember, that all this happened over twenty years ago and many improvements will have been made during that time.

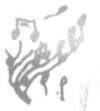

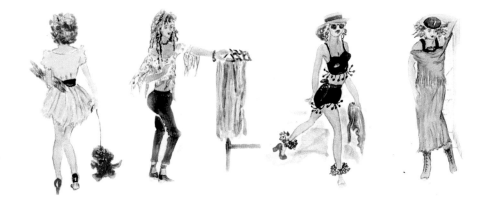

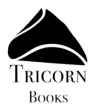

TRICORN

BOOKS